Mirrors in the Brain—How Our Minds Share Actions and Emotions

Mirrors in the Brain—How Our Minds Share Actions and Emotions

Giacomo Rizzolatti,
Corrado Sinigaglia

Translated by

Frances Anderson

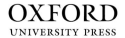
OXFORD
UNIVERSITY PRESS

OXFORD

UNIVERSITY PRESS

Great Clarendon Street, Oxford OX2 6DP

Oxford University Press is a department of the University of Oxford.
It furthers the University's objective of excellence in research, scholarship,
and education by publishing worldwide in

Oxford New York

Auckland Cape Town Dar es Salaam Hong Kong Karachi
Kuala Lumpur Madrid Melbourne Mexico City Nairobi
New Delhi Shanghai Taipei Toronto

With offices in

Argentina Austria Brazil Chile Czech Republic France Greece
Guatemala Hungary Italy Japan Poland Portugal
Singapore South Korea Switzerland Thailand Turkey Ukraine Vietnam

Oxford is a registered trade mark of Oxford University Press
in the UK and in certain other countries

Published in the United States
by Oxford University Press Inc., New York

© Raffaello Cortina Editore 2006

The translation of this work has been funded by SEPS
SEGRETARIATO EUROPEO PER LE PUBBLICAZIONI SCIENTIFICHE

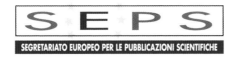

Via Val d'Aposa 7 - 40123 Bologna - Italy
tel +39 051 271992 - fax +39 051 265983
seps@alma.unibo.it - www.seps.it

The moral rights of the author have been asserted
Database right Oxford University Press (maker)

First published (Italian) 2006
First published (English) 2008

A catalogue record for this title is available from the British Library
Data available

Typeset by Cepha Imaging Private Ltd., Bangalore, India
Printed in China
on acid-free paper through
Asia Pacific Offset

1005712657

ISBN 978–0–19–921798–4

10 9 8 7 6 5 4 3 2

Contents

Acknowledgements

First, we would like to thank Giulio Giorello for having believed in this book; without his support, bringing this project to fruition would have been most arduous.

Much of the research and the findings described in this book are the result of years of study carried out at the University of Parma, in which many friends and colleagues have actively participated. Massimo Matelli, Maurizio Gentilucci, and Giuseppe Luppino have contributed enormously to the definition of the multiple cortical motor areas and the study of their functions. Luciano Fadiga, Leonardo Fogassi, and Vittorio Gallese have actively participated in the discovery of the surprising properties of the mirror neurons from the very beginning. Michael Arbib, Marc Jeannerod, and Hideo Sakata have played a key role in the elaboration of the theory presented in this book. Sincere thanks are due to Scott Grafton, Marco Iacoboni, Giovanni Buccino, and the brain imaging group of Milan directed by Ferruccio Fazio, for their help with innumerable PET and fMRI experiments. Laila Craighero, Pier Francesco Ferrari, Christian Keysers, and Maria Alessandra Umiltà have contributed with extensive experimental work: our sincere thanks goes to them and all the other members, past and present, of the Parma team.

We are grateful to Claudio Bartocci, Giorgio Bertolotti, Antonio Cilluffo, Gabriella Morandi, and Stefano Moriggi for reading parts of the manuscript and for their valuable comments and suggestions. Domenico Mallamo helped us with the illustrations and diagrams.

Finally, we wish to express our sincere appreciation to Mariella Agostinelli for the passion and proficiency she dedicated to each phase of the project, to Raffaella Voi and Giorgio Catalano for their patience and invaluable editorial assistance, and to Frances Anderson for translating this work with utmost care and enthusiasm.

Preface

In an interview some time ago, the great theatrical director, Peter Brook commented that with the discovery of mirror neurons, neuroscience had finally started to understand what has long been common knowledge in the theatre: the actor's efforts would be in vain if he were not able to surmount all cultural and linguistic barriers and share his bodily sounds and movements with the spectators, who thus actively contribute to the event and become one with the players on the stage. This sharing is the basis on which the theatre evolves and revolves, and mirror neurons, which become active both when an individual executes an act and when he observes it being executed by others, now provide this sharing with a biological explanation.

Brook's mention of mirror neurons evidences the enormous interest their unexpected properties have roused in fields other than neurophysiology. Artists, psychologists, pedagogues, sociologists, anthropologists, and many others have been held in thrall by mirror neurons, but probably only a few know the story of their discovery and the experimental research and theoretical assumptions that made it possible; fewer still imagine the implications that this discovery will have on how we perceive and understand the architecture and the functioning of the brain.

This, then, is the topic of this book. It starts with an analysis of certain day-to-day gestures —such as reaching for an object and grasping it with the hand, carrying food to the mouth—the importance of which we tend to underestimate just because they are so routine. For many years, too, neuroscience (and other disciplines) relegated the *motor system*, which plays the leading role behind these gestures, to that of a mere extra.

For decades the concept that the motor areas of the cerebral cortex were destined to carry out merely executive tasks reigned supreme; it was thought that these were completely without any effective perceptive, let alone cognitive, value. In this view, the elaboration of the diverse sensorial input and the individuation of the neural substrate of the cognitive processes linked to the production of intentions, beliefs, and desires constituted the greatest difficulties in explaining our motor behaviour. Once it has been recognized that the brain is able to select the flow of information coming from the outside and integrate it with mental representations generated more or less automatically within, the problems inherent to movement would be reduced to the mechanics of its execution—according to the classical pattern: perception $\rightarrow$ cognition $\rightarrow$ movement.

This pattern was perfectly satisfactory as long as an oversimplified view of the motor system prevailed. Today, however, this view has changed. We know that not only is this system composed of a mosaic of frontal and parietal areas that are very closely linked to the visual, auditory, and tactile areas, but it is also endowed with functional properties that are much more complex than was previously thought. In particular it has been discovered that in certain areas there are neurons that become active in response to goal-directed motor acts (such as grasping, holding, manipulating, etc.) and not just to simple movements; not only, they also respond selectively to the shapes and sizes of objects both when we interact with them and also when we just observe them. These neurons appear to be able to discriminate sensorial information, coding it on the basis of the range of potential acts offered, independently of whether they subsequently evolve into a concrete action.

If we take a look at the mechanisms underlying the workings of the brain, it is clear just how abstract are those explanations customarily given to our behaviour, which tend to separate our intentional acts from the pure physical movement required to execute them. Just as abstract, in fact, as many of the experiments usually carried out to record neuron activity and in which animals, monkeys for example, are regarded as little robots programmed to perform rigidly specified tasks. If, on the other hand, neuron activity is recorded in an ethological context, leaving the animal free to take the food and objects offered as it likes, then it becomes clear that at the cortical level the motor system is not just involved with single movements but with actions. Think about it; the same is just as true for humans: we very rarely move our arms, hands, and mouth without a goal; there is usually an object to be reached, grasped, or bitten into.

These acts, insofar as they are *goal-directed* and *not merely movements*, provide the basis for our experience of our surroundings and endow objects with the immediate meaning they hold for us. That rigid divide between perceptive, motor, and cognitive processes is to a great extent artificial; not only does perception appear to be embedded in the dynamics of action, becoming much more composite than used to be thought in the past, but *the acting brain* is also and above all *a brain that understands*. As we will see, this is a pragmatic, pre-conceptual, and pre-linguistic form of understanding, but is no less important for that, because it lies at the base of many of our celebrated cognitive abilities.

This type of understanding is also reflected in the activation of the mirror neurons. These were discovered at the beginning of the 1990s and show how recognition of the actions of others, and even of their intentions, depends first of all on our motor repertoire. From elementary acts such as grasping to the more sophisticated that require particular skills such as playing a sonata on a pianoforte or executing complicated dance steps, the mirror neurons allow our brain to match the movements we observe to the movements we ourselves can perform, and so to appreciate their meaning. Without a mirror mechanism we would still have our sensory representation, a 'pictorial' depiction of the behaviour of others, but we would not know what they were really doing. Certainly, we could use our higher cognitive faculties to reflect on what we have perceived and infer the intentions, expectations, or motivations of others that would provide us with a reason for their acts, but our brain is able to understand these latter immediately on the basis of our motor competencies alone, without the need of any kind of reasoning.

It would seem therefore that the mirror neuron system is indispensable to that sharing of experience which is at the root of our capacity to act as individuals but also as members of a society. Forms of imitation, both simple and complex, of learning, of verbal and gestural communication, presuppose the activation of specific mirror circuits. Moreover, our capacity to appreciate the emotional reactions of others is correlated to a particular group of areas that are characterized by mirror properties. Emotions, like actions, are immediately shared; the perception of pain or grief, or of disgust experienced by others, activates the same areas of the cerebral cortex that are involved when we experience these emotions ourselves.

This shows how strong and deeply rooted is the bond that ties us to others, or in other words, how bizarre it would be to conceive of an *I* without an *us*. As Peter Brook reminds us, the players on the stage overcome all linguistic and cultural barriers to encompass the spectators in a shared experience of actions and emotions. The study of mirror neurons appears to offer, for the first time, a unitary experimental and theoretical framework within which to decipher this form of shared participation that the theatre provides and which is fundamentally the basis of our common experience.

CHAPTER 1

The motor system

A cup of coffee

Let us start with a practical example. What could be simpler than picking up a cup of coffee? Yet this simple gesture requires a plethora of processes so closely interconnected that at first glance it is difficult to distinguish one from another. First of all we must identify the cup from the various objects vying for our attention; to do this we must swivel our head and eyes so that the image of the cup will land on our fovea where visual acuity is at its height and examine its various aspects (shape, orientation of the handle, colour, and so on). Then to actually pick the cup up, we have to assess its exact location with respect to our body, and only when this has been done can we extend a hand towards it, while at the same time sizing it up, so to speak, in order to grasp it in the most appropriate manner.

The cup itself supplies information relative to *geometrical properties* and *ways of grasping*: it is up to us to decide how to act on this information, to choose the prehension we find most suitable or to which we are most accustomed. Although we may not always be conscious of these preliminaries, our fingers start to curl and the palm of our hand to curve, assuming a shape that will mould to the geometrical properties of the part of the cup we are aiming at even before we make contact with it. As soon as we touch the cup, the hand receives information from our skin, joints, and muscles, which enables us to perfect the grasp and carry the cup to the mouth.

So, behind this simple gesture of picking up a cup of coffee lies a complex intertwining of sensations (visual, tactile, olfactory, proprioceptive), motivational connections, body arrangements, and motor performance, not to speak of postural adjustments—which anticipate the execution of each of these movements and their consequences and guarantee the required control over the body's dynamic balance—and the role played by the learning process and the know-how we have acquired in identifying, localizing, reaching for, and grasping objects in general. All these factors interact more or less harmonically with each other and with the objects which populate our world.

Now we have described, very briefly, the complexity of the processes involved in picking up a cup of coffee, but what happens when we pass into the realm of neurophysiology? Are we to expect that these processes are connected to cortical circuits that are quite distinct from an anatomical and functional point of view? When we pick up that cup of coffee, which of our neural systems are involved at cortical level? How do they interact?

The organization of the frontal motor areas

It may surprise many of our readers that such an everyday gesture should be used to talk about neuroscience, not to mention the cognitive sciences, but over the last twenty years analyses of the neural mechanisms underlying elementary acts such as grasping (and the numerous other acts so common in our daily lives) have made us take a second look at many key aspects of the traditional view of how the brain works, particularly with regard to the organization of the motor system and its functional relations with the other systems (such as, but not only, the sensorial systems).

It has long been thought that sensory, perceptive, and motor mechanisms were situated in clearly distinct cortical areas: on one side, there were the *sensory areas*, including the visual areas located in the occipital lobe, the somatosensory areas in the postcentral gyrus, the auditory areas in the superior temporal gyrus, and so on, while on the other the *motor areas* were to be found in the posterior region of the frontal lobe, also known as the *agranular frontal cortex*. According to this view, vast cortical regions—often defined as the *associative areas*—were located between the sensory and motor areas; it was thought that in those associative areas, particularly in the temporo-parietal regions, information from the various sensory areas was assembled and objectual and spatial percepts formed for dispatch to the motor areas for organization into movement (Figure 1.1).

According to this model, when we pick up an object with our hands the brain implements a number of serially organized processes, sending the information which arrives from the sensory areas to the associative areas for integration, and then transmitting the resulting data to the motor cortex to activate the appropriate movements.

The role of the motor system would therefore be peripheral and almost exclusively executive, as can be seen from the functional maps that appear in practically all neurology and neuroscience manuals. Examples of these are Clinton Woolsey's classic *simiunculus* and Wilder Penfield's equally classic *homunculus* (Figure 1.2), obtained during the twentieth century by electrical stimulation by macro-electrodes placed on the surface of the motor cortex of monkeys (*simiunculus*)

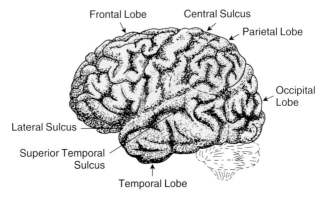

Fig. 1.1 Lateral view of the human cortex. The occipital lobe and the part of the temporal lobe that is situated below the temporal sulcus (the 'inferotemporal' lobe) have visual functions. The primary auditory areas are buried within the lateral sulcus, also known as the fissure of Silvius (Silvian fissure). The superior temporal gyrus (the cortex above the superior temporal sulcus) has mostly auditory functions. The superior temporal sulcus conceals both higher-order visual areas and polymodal areas (areas in which visual, auditory and somatic modalities converge). The anterior portion of the parietal lobe contains areas responsive to tactile and proprioceptive stimuli, while the posterior portion houses areas with functions traditionally classified as associative. The posterior section of the frontal lobe contains the motor areas, while the anterior section (the 'prefrontal' lobe) contains areas with cognitive functions.

and of humans (*homunculus*).[1] Both distinguished two motor areas: the primary motor area (MI) and the supplementary motor area (SMA, which is also sometimes indicated as MII), characterized by a complete representation of movements— more detailed in MI, somewhat sketchy in SMA.

These maps were not however in total accord with the cytoarchitectonic organization of the posterior region of the

---

[1]   Woolsey *et al.* (1952); Woolsey (1958); Penfield and Rasmussen (1950).

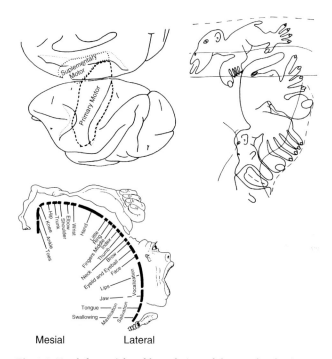

Mesial   Lateral

Fig. 1.2 Top left: mesial and lateral view of the monkey brain. The dashed lines delimit the primary and the supplementary motor areas as they were mapped in classical neurology. Top right: the *simiunculi* of Clinton Woolsey. The two *simiunculi* schematically illustrate the representation of movements in the primary and supplementary motor cortices. Bottom left: Wilder Penfield's motor *homunculus*.

frontal lobe (motor cortex) in primates described by Korbinian Brodmann[2] at the beginning of the twentieth century. Brodmann divided this region of the frontal lobe into two distinct areas (areas 4 and 6) on the basis of the distribution of pyramidal cells in the V cortical layer (Figure 1.3).

---

[2] Brodmann (1909).

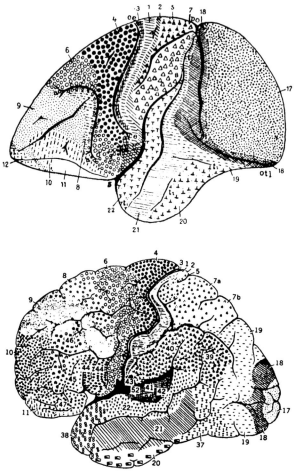

Fig. 1.3 Cytoarchitectonic maps of the monkey (*Cercopithecus aethiops*) and human cortices (left and right, respectively). These maps were drawn by Brodmann using a histological method that stains the cell bodies (method of Nissl). This method allows one to recognize a series of cortical areas distinguished by the number (normally six) and size of their layers, the number of neurons they contain, and the distribution of the fundamental types of cortical neurons (pyramidal, stellar or gtanular, and fusiform

The MI in fact included all of area 4 and most of area 6 on the lateral surface of the hemisphere, while the SMA coincided with the part of area 6 located on the mesial surface. Woolsey, in an attempt to explain this inconsistency, suggested that the cytoarchitectonic discrepancy between areas 4 and 6 did not embody a functional distinction, but simply a diverse somatotopic representation. Thus movements of the hand, mouth, and foot (distal movements) would be localized in area 4, while area 6 would be the site

----

neurons). These maps show that monkey and human cortices have several basic similarities: both have the same main sulci (the central sulcus, lateral sulcus, superior temporal sulcus), and, with a few exceptions, the same cytoarchitectonic areas. But there are also a number of important differences: for example, the parietotemporal occipital region is much more extensive in man than in the monkey. This has caused a shift in the visual areas, which, in the human cortex, occupy the mesial face of the hemisphere, while in the monkey they take up a large portion of the caudal pole of the brain hemispheres on the lateral surface (area 17). In addition, in humans the frontal lobe is significantly enlarged. Monkeys, on the other hand, have a sulcus that is not present in humans, the arcuate sulcus, which divides the frontal lobe into two portions that differ both cytoarchitectonically and functionally. The posterior portion, formed by areas 4 and 6, is characterized by an almost total absence of granules and the fact that the fourth layer (the internal granular layer) is absent (hence the term agranular cortex). Although macroscopic examinations in humans do not show such a well-defined subdivision of the frontal lobe, cytoarchitectonic studies and functional analyses indicate that also in humans it is possible to distinguish, in this lobe, between a posterior and an anterior part, the former (consisting of areas 4 and 6) being concerned primarily with motor activities, while the latter (frequently referred to as the prefrontal lobe) is involved in cognitive functions.

of arm and leg movements (proximal movements) and movements of the trunk (axial movements).

Although this was considered by many to be an *ad hoc* solution, and as such received a fair amount of criticism, the general concept of the two *simiunculi* was regarded as one of the key stones of neurology for many years. There were at least two reasons for this: in the first place, it provide a direct explanation, easily applicable from the clinical point of view, to the problem of localization of movements in the motor cortex; second, it reflects the theory that is as widespread today as it was in the past, of the functional unity of the motor cortex, considered to be the arrival point for the sensorial information processed by the associative areas, totally devoid of any perceptive or cognitive role.

In the words of Elwood Henneman, such a system would exist in the brain only 'to translate thought and sensation into movement'.[3] The question of course, is *how* and *when* such translation takes place. In other words, when do *thought* and *sensation* cease to be such and become *movement*? Henneman added that 'at the present the initial steps of this process lie beyond analysis'.[4] However, only a few years after that 'present' (1984), it became clear that not only is the motor system connected anatomically to the cortical areas responsible for the cerebral activity involved in '*thought and sensation*', but it also has a plurality of functions that are not compatible with the concept of a sole, purely executive map.

Far from being organized in just two areas (MI and SMA), the cortical motor system is formed by a constellation of various areas.[5] A comparison of the current view of the

---

[3]   Henneman (1984, p. 670).
[4]   Ibidem.
[5]   Matelli *et al.* (1985; 1991); Petrides and Pandya (1997).

anatomic-functional parcellation of the agranular cortex as illustrated in Figure 1.4 with the maps shown in Figures 1.2 and 1.3, shows how, contrary to Woolsey's hypothesis, the primary motor cortex (MI, which we will now refer to as F1) coincides with Brodmann's area 4. Area 6, on the other

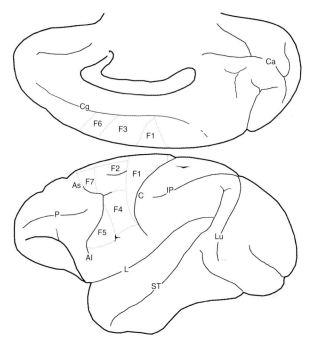

Fig. 1.4 Mesial and lateral view of the monkey brain showing the anatomo-functional parcellation of the frontal motor cortex. The letter F followed by an Arabic number indicates the areas of the frontal agranular cortex. This nomenclature is derived from that used by von Economo, Koskinas, 1925, to classify the areas of the human cortex. Other abbreviations used: Ai inferior arcuate sulcus, As superior arcuate sulcus, C central sulcus, Ca calcarine fissure, Cg cingulate sulcus, IP intraparietal sulcus, L lateral fissure or fissure of Silvius, Lu lunate sulcus, P main sulcus, ST superior temporal sulcus.

hand, is subdivided into three main regions (*mesial, dorsal,* and *ventral*), which in turn are subdivided into rostral (anterior) and caudal (posterior) parts: the *mesial region* is formed by two areas, F3 (SMA) and F6 (pre-SMA); the *dorsal region* (the premotor dorsal cortex) by F2 (known as PMd) and F7 (pre-PMd) while F4 and F5 form the *ventral region* (the premotor ventral cortex, PMv).

The use of more sophisticated electrophysiological techniques—in which microelectrodes capable of stimulating small groups of projection neurons (intracortical microstimulation) are inserted in the cortex—has shown that the motor cortex contains a number of maps, which are functionally distinct one from another and which are localized in the areas listed above. It has been discovered that, with regard to the mesial region of area 6, F3 can be electrically stimulated with low intensity currents and contains a complete representation of body movements, while area F6 can only be stimulated by higher intensity currents and produces only slow and complex brachial motor movements. In the dorsal region, area F2 can be stimulated electrically and has a rough somatotopic organization (with a leg and an arm representation located dorsal and ventral to the superior precentral dimple, respectively); area F7, on the other hand, is not particularly responsive to electrical stimuli and its functional properties are little known. Finally, with regard to the ventral region, both areas F4 and F5 respond to electrical stimulation, but while the motor representations of the former regard the arms, neck, and movements of the face, those of the latter predominantly involve the hands and the mouth.

Even more significant from a functional point of view are the data obtained from the recordings of single neurons. These have shown how the various areas of the motor cortex respond in different ways to sensory stimuli and they also reveal significant dissimilarities during active movements. The subdivision of the motor cortex into two areas (MI, SMA) would therefore seem too simplistic and if we do not want to reject Woolsey's *simiunculi* theory outright, then we must at least adjust it slightly, substituting the classic dual representation with a multiple somatotopic account. Moreover, the discovery that the anatomic–functional structure of the agranular frontal cortex is more complex than was thought in the past, helps to overcome the apparent dichotomy between the motor system on the one hand and the sensory systems (visual, auditory, olfactory, somatosensory, etc.) on the other.

There is a general consensus that the retina and the cochlear have multiple representations in the cerebral cortex; the same is true for the various cytoarchitectonic areas that contain independent somatosensory representations. Why therefore should we be surprised if the motor cortex reveals an analogous multiplicity of distinct representations? The problem is rather to establish, given such anatomical and functional abundance, how the various areas perform in the organization and control of movement. Do they operate in a hierarchy or in parallel? Is their sphere of action limited to the functions normally assigned to them or do they also embrace other functions traditionally reserved for the 'associative' areas, which are crucial for the 'translation' of sensory information into motor commands?

The parietofrontal circuits

A complete understanding of the nature and scope of the motor cortex system requires more than just an identification of the various pieces that make up the mosaic of the anatomically and functionally distinct areas of the agranular cortex. We also have to consider their connections with the other motor areas (*the intrinsic connections*), those which have the cortical areas outside the agranular frontal cortex (*the extrinsic connections*) as well as the organization of their projections to the subcortical centres and the spinal cord (*the descending connections*).

We now know that there is a considerable difference between the motor areas situated in the posterior sector of the agranular frontal cortex (F2–F5) and the anterior motor areas (F6–F7). The former are directly connected with F1 and appear to be linked together somatotopically, while the latter do not project into F1 but have strong connections with the other motor areas.[6] We find a similar subdivision at the level of the descending projections. F1, F2, F3, and parts of F4 and F5 give rise to the corticospinal tract, but neither F6 nor F7 are actually connected to the spinal cord; they project out to other sectors of the brainstem, which means that unlike the posterior areas they can only control movement indirectly, through their subcortical relays.[7]

It is interesting to note that the fibres which originate from F1 terminate in the intermediate section of the spinal cord and in the lamina in which the motor neurons are located, while those which descend from the other motor areas (F2–F5) end almost exclusively in the intermediate region of the spinal cord. This anatomic difference produces a diversity in function: the projections of F2, F3, F4, and F5 activate

---

[6] See Matsumara and Kubota (1979); Muakkassa and Strick (1979); Matelli *et al.* (1986); Lupino *et al.* (1993).

[7] Further information can be obtained from Keizer and Kuypers (1989); He *et al.* (1993; 1995); Galea and Darian-Smith (1994); Rizzolatti and Luppino (2001).

preformed medullar circuits, which determine the overall frame of movement; the projections of F1, on the other hand, as they end directly on the motor neurons, break hardwired synergies and are responsible for the fine morphology of movement.

With regard to the *extrinsic connections*, the agranular frontal cortex areas receive cortical afferents from three principal regions: the prefrontal lobe, the cingulate cortex, and the parietal lobe (the primary somatosensory cortex, or SI, and the posterior parietal cortex).

It is generally accepted that the *prefrontal lobe* plays a significant role in the so-called higher order functions, such as the working memory and temporal action planning. It has also often been attributed with coherency of intention: it is well known that people with prefrontal lesions have difficulty in acting on their intentions and are easily distracted.[8] This has given rise to the belief that the prefrontal regions house the neural substrate where the intentions which precede and guide our actions are formed.

Little is known about the *cingulate cortex*; however, it is widely held that this region is involved in the processing of motivational and emotional information which are the basis of our intentions and influence the course of our actions.

Finally, as far as the *posterior parietal lobe* is concerned, a more detailed anatomical description is required, as without this, it would not be possible to fully understand the possible functions of the various motor circuits.

In primates, the posterior parietal lobe is divided into two main sectors by one of the oldest sulcus in evolutionary terms: the intraparietal sulcus (IP). These sectors are the superior parietal lobe (SPL) and the inferior parietal lobe (IPL), both

---

[8] See Fuster (1989).

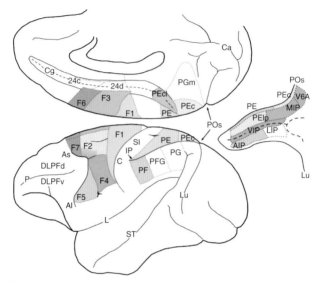

Fig. 1.5 Mesial and lateral view of the monkey brain. The motor cortex and of the posterior parietal cortex are subdivided in a series of anatomical and functional areas. The areas of the posterior parietal cortex are designated by the letter P followed by one or more letters. The drawing on the right shows the areas buried in the intraparietal sulcus (IP): AIP anterior intraparietal area, LIP lateral intraparietal area, MIP medial intraparietal area, PEIp intraparietal PE area, VIP ventral intraparietal area. Other abbreviations used: Cg cingulate sulcus, DLPFd dorsal dorsolateral prefrontal cortex; DLPFv ventral dorsolateral prefrontal cortex, SI primary somatosensory cortex, Pos parieto-occipital sulcus. For abbreviations other than those listed above refer to Fig. 1.4 (Luppino, Rizzolatti, 2000).

of which are formed by a vast number of independent areas, whose function would appear to be to process particular aspects of sensory information and which are connected to specific effectors (Figure 1.5). Some of these areas are linked to somatosensory modalities, others to visual modalities, and some to both.[9]

The posterior parietal cortex presents a rich parcellation analogous to that found in the motor cortex. It is important to note that neural activity has been observed in connection with motor acts in the posterior parietal regions, which have long been classified as *associative* regions.[10] Therefore, if the definition of *motor* neurons as neurons connected with movement is correct, the posterior parietal cortex must be considered part of the cortical motor system. This is substantiated by the fact that from an anatomical point of view the frontal parietal connections show a high level of specificity, which results in a series of anatomically segregated circuits. The functional correlate of this situation is that each of these circuits appears to be involved in a particular sensory–motor transformation or, in other words, in a particular 'translation' of a sensory stimulus into a motor stimulus.

Let us return briefly to the frontal motor areas. We have seen how these are divided into posterior (F1–F5) and anterior (F6 and F7) areas. The following diagrams show how such a subdivision is also applicable to their *extrinsic connections*. The posterior motor areas receive their principal cortical afferents from the parietal lobe (Figure 1.6);

---

[9] See Colby *et al.* (1988); Colby and Duhamel (1991); Tanné *et al.* (1995); Lacquaniti *et al.* (1995); Caminiti *et al.* (1996); Rizzolatti *et al.* (1997); Wise *et al.* (1997).

[10] See Mountcastle *et al.* (1975); Hyvärinen (1981); Andersen (1987); Sakata *et al.* (1995).

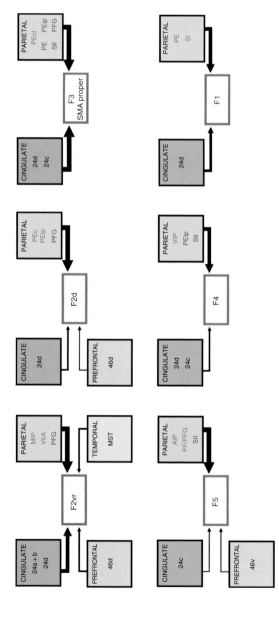

Fig. 1.6 Schematic representation of the extrinsic afferent connections of the posterior motor areas. The strength of the connections is indicated by the thickness of the arrows. The parietal areas that send the main motor input to a given motor area are indicated in red print, those that are the source of minor projections are indicated in black. (Rizzolatti, Luppino, 2001).

the anterior motor areas, on the other hand, receive theirs from the prefrontal cortex and the cingulate cortex (Figure 1.7).

It has therefore to be concluded that the two types of motor area have different functions. The posterior areas receive a wealth of sensory information from the parietal lobe, which is then used to organize and control movement. This information is elaborated by parallel processes in which each circuit is involved in specific sensory–motor transformations; for example, some circuits analyse somatosensory information to specify the body parts involved in controlling limb movement, others use visual information to code our surrounding space, to reach for objects, or move the hand in an appropriate manner. The anterior areas, on the contrary, receive little sensory information and so it is highly unlikely that they play a significant role in the sensory–motor transformation process. However they do receive higher order cognitive information related to long-term motor plans or to motivations and this lends plausibility to the hypothesis that these areas have mainly control functions, determining when and under which circumstances the potential motor acts selected by the posterior areas must be transformed into an effective act.[11]

An initial conclusion

This brief introduction to the organization of the cortical areas and their connections shows how, over the past twenty years, experimental data have significantly changed the original

---

[11]   For greater detail, see Rizzolatti *et al.* (1998).

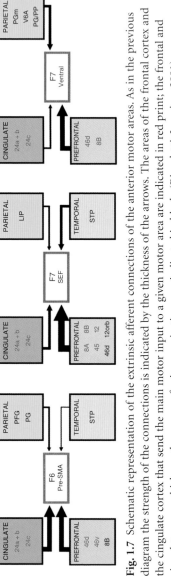

Fig. 1.7 Schematic representation of the extrinsic afferent connections of the anterior motor areas. As in the previous diagram the strength of the connections is indicated by the thickness of the arrows. The areas of the frontal cortex and the cingulate cortex that send the main motor input to a given motor area are indicated in red print; the frontal and cingulate areas which are the source of minor projections are indicated in black. (Rizzolatti, Luppino, 2001).

view of the motor system which dominated the scene in physiology and the neurosciences for many years. The agranular frontal cortex and the posterior parietal cortex are composed of a mosaic of regions which are strongly inter-connected but are anatomically and functionally distinct, forming circuits which work in parallel and integrate the sensory and motor information relative to specific effectors. The same holds true for the circuits which involve the prefrontal and cingulate cortices, which are responsible for forming intentions, long-term planning, and deciding the appropriate time at which to act.

In the light of these findings a number of assumptions are no longer adequate and this is true not only for the classic maps drawn up on the lines traced by Woolsey and Penfield. For example, the assumption widely held in the past and still cited today that the sensory, perceptive, and motor functions are housed in distinct and separate regions would appear to be an oversimplification. In fact, the vast number of structures and functions found to belong to the motor system makes it increasingly evident that its role cannot be that of a passive executor of commands originating elsewhere.

Besides, when the role of motor system was considered as being limited to the production of movement, there was no way of understanding the initial phases of that process, i.e. of understanding 'how' and 'where' the sensory information, the intentions, motivations, etc. were 'translated' into appropriate motor events. At that point, falling back on the associative areas was more an indication of the existence of the problem rather than the solution itself. One of the first questions that comes to mind, in fact, is which mechanisms were used to transform the 'associations' into motor input?

Significant changes to the traditional view were brought about by the discovery that the areas of the posterior parietal cortex (traditionally labelled as 'associative'), not only receive strong afferents from the sensory areas but also possess motor properties that are analogous to those of the agranular frontal cortex, to the extent that together they actually form highly specialized intracortical circuits. This showed that, far from being peripheral to and isolated from the rest of the cerebral activity, the motor system is made up of a complex web of cortical areas that are anatomically and functionally different and contribute to produce those sensory–motor translations (or, more precisely, transformations) required to individuate and locate objects and implement the movements required to execute the acts that compose our daily lives. Moreover, the fact that sensory and motor information have a common format characterized by specific fronto-parietal circuits would suggest that the motor system has a number of other functions, over and above organizing our motor behaviour. These include certain processes that are normally considered as being higher order and therefore attributed to cognitive systems; for example, the perception and recognition of actions carried out by others, imitation, and gestural and vocal communication; it may well be that the primary neural substrate of these processes lies in the motor system.

We will discuss these topics in greater detail in the following chapters, but now it is time to have that cup of coffee.

CHAPTER 2

The acting brain

Movements and motor acts

In the first chapter we have seen that the act of picking up an object, our cup of coffee for example, is a combination of two processes, *reaching* and *grasping*, which, though independent, are inter-coordinated. It is commonly thought that the former precedes the latter, but this is not so. Recordings of the movements of the arm and hand show that these processes start and proceed in parallel. The arm moves towards the cup and contemporaneously the hand assumes the shape necessary to grasp it.

Let us take a closer look at the latter process. In order for the hand to actually *grasp* an object, the brain has to: (1) possess a mechanism which transforms the sensory information relative to the geometrical properties (the 'intrinsic properties') of the object to be grasped into an appropriate shaping of the fingers; (2) be able to control the movements of the hand, particularly of the fingers, to execute the actual grasping.

It has been known for some time now that this latter function requires the involvement of the primary motor cortex (F1), which, in virtue of its direct connections with the motor neurons of the spinal cord, is the only area which controls isolated movements of the fingers (i.e. movements which are not part of hardwired synergies). Damage to F1 results in flaccidity and a loss of strength and destroys the capacity of moving the fingers independently.[1]

However, F1 does not have direct access to visual information; moreover the neurons in this area which do respond to visual stimuli (and they are very few) are not able to transform the geometrical properties of objects into the appropriate motor patterns. These transformations are essential for acts such as grasping, and now we know that they are done by area F5.

We have already mentioned that F5 contains motor representations of the hand and mouth which partially overlap each other. One of the techniques most frequently used to individuate the functions of this area, as of other cortical areas, consists in recording the activity of single neurons and correlating it with motor behaviour in animals. There are two very different ways of doing this: either the neuron activity can be recorded during experiments in which the animal performs only movements which it has been trained to make[2] and which have been previously established by the experimenter or while it is performing a wide range of spontaneous movements in as natural a context as possible.

Although the second approach may appear somewhat subjective, it does have a number of significant advantages. When neurons are studied during fixed and stereotypical movements, only the properties relative to the motor activities chosen *a priori* by the experimenter will emerge, thus eliminating the possibility of discovering unexpected

---

[1] See, for example, Schieber and Poliakov (1998); Fogassi *et al.* (2001); a review of preceding literature can be found in Porter and Lemon (1993).

[2] See, for example, Evarts *et al.*; Poliakov (1984); Weinrich and Wise (2001).

aspects of the neural organization. On the other hand, if the recordings are done in a more natural context in which, for instance, the monkey is allowed to pick up different types of objects, the study is less susceptible to preconceived notions which often run the risk of degenerating into pure prejudice. In addition there is always the possibility of discovering new and unexpected functionalities.

It is not surprising, therefore, that it was a study using this approach that revealed an unforeseen property of area F5: the majority of its neurons code *motor acts* (i.e. goal-directed movements) and not *individual movements*.[3] In fact, many F5 neurons discharge when the monkey performs a motor act, for example when it grasps a piece of food, irrespective of whether it uses its right or left hand or even its mouth to do so. It has also been seen that in many cases, a particular movement that activates a neuron during a specific motor act does not do so during other seemingly related acts; for example, bending the index finger triggers a neuron when grasping, but not when scratching. Therefore the activity of these neurons cannot be adequately described in terms of pure movement, but taking the efficacy of the motor act as the fundamental criterion of classification they can be sub-divided into specific categories, of which the most common are 'grasping-with-the-hand-and-the-mouth', 'grasping-with-the-hand', 'holding', 'tearing', 'manipulating', and so on.

Figure 2.1 illustrates the behaviour of a typical 'grasping-with-the-hand-and-the-mouth' neuron, which was seen to fire when the animal picked up a morsel of food with its mouth (A), with the contralateral hand (B), and the ipsilateral hand (C). The neuron did not respond in any way

---

[3] Rizzolatti and Gentilucci (1988); Rizzolatti *et al.* (1988).

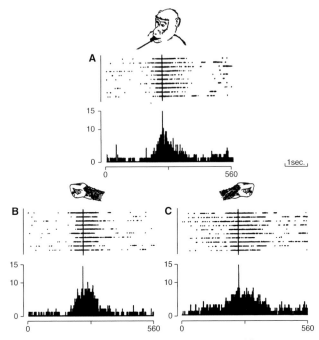

Fig. 2.1 A "grasping-with-the-hand-and-the-mouth" F5 neuron. The panels show the activity of the neuron when the monkey grasps a piece of food with its mouth (A), with the controlateral hand (B), and the ipsilateral hand (C). Rasters and histograms are aligned with the instant in which the monkey touches the food. The histograms represent the average of ten trials. The *abscissa* shows the time expressed in bin (1 bin = 10 ms), while the ordinate shows the spikes/bin ratio. (Adapted from Rizzolatti et al., 1988.)

to the opening and closing of the mouth caused by stimuli other than food such as emotional stimuli, nor did it respond when the animal extended its arm without grasping the food or simply to push away objects which were disturbing it. To recap these findings, movements of the mouth or hands performed during acts other than grasping did not trigger the neuron, in spite of the fact that the same muscles are involved; vice versa, the neuron did respond when the monkey carried out different movements with the same goal, i.e. that of getting food.

Most F5 neurons, irrespective of their category, also code the shape the hand has to adopt to execute the act in question, so we find neurons which become active when the monkey uses the precision grip (which is characterized by index–thumb opposition and is particularly useful for picking up small objects); others which discharge when the monkey uses all the fingers of its hand to grasp the object (this grip is normally used for medium-sized objects); finally others, which are rather rare, that fire during whole hand prehension, also known as prehension force, used for large objects. The neurons that code the gripping of a sphere, for example, which requires whole hand prehension (pressure exerted by all the fingers), are different to those which code the gripping of a cylinder, for which the pressure of the thumb is not necessary.[4]

Not only are F5 neurons specific to certain types of prehension, they also discharge at different phases of the motor act. For example, in the case of grasping with the hand, approximately one-third of the neurons start to fire while the fingers are being flexed, while the remaining two-thirds fire prior to the flexing and continue to discharge almost until the grip is fully achieved. Of these latter neurons, approximately 50% discharge while the fingers are being extended, while the other half fire before any observable distal movement commences. This constitutes

---

[4] Jeannerod *et al.* (1995).

further evidence that F5 neurons respond selectively to motor acts and not to individual movements. In fact, with the exception of those which discharge exclusively in the final phase of the grasping process, the other F5 neurons (which account for approximately 70% of the total) fire both while the fingers are being extended (pre-shaping of the prehension) and flexed (the actual grip). It is therefore rather difficult to attribute their activation to any particular movement, whether it be the extending or the flexing of the fingers.[5]

Visuo-motor properties

The *motor* properties that have been described in the preceding section are typical of F5 neurons. However, from the earliest studies on the subject it has been seen that a portion of these neurons respond selectively also to visual stimuli.[6] An experimental paradigm, designed to disentangle the visual from the motor responses and throw light on their characteristics, was therefore devised to further investigate the visuo-motor functions of the F5 neurons.

In this experiment, which was conducted by Akira Murata and his colleagues[7], a monkey was seated in front of a box containing six solid objects of different geometric shapes and sizes (a plate, a ring, a cube, a cylinder, a cone, and a sphere). These objects were shown to the monkey one at a time and always in the same central position. The experiment consisted of three conditions: (A) grasping the object in the light; (B) grasping the object in the dark;

---

[5] Rizzolatti and Gentilucci (1988).
[6] See, for example, Rizzolatti *et al.* (1988).
[7] Murata *et al.* (1997). See also Rizzolatti *et al.* (2000); Gallese (2000).

and (C) object fixation. In the first condition, a spot of red light from a red/green light-emitting diode (LED) was projected onto the object which however was not visible. The animal had to stare at this spot of light, and then press a key which illuminated the box and its contents. The red LED then turned green, at which point the monkey had to release the key and grasp the object. In the second condition, the animal initially grasped the object after seeing it; subsequently the light was extinguished and the following trials were conducted in the dark. In this condition, therefore, the monkey was no longer able to rely on sight, but had to fall back on its previous knowledge of the localization and characteristics of the object. In the third condition, which to all effects and purposes replicated the first, when the red LED turned to green the monkey had to release the key and merely fixate the object without grasping it.

The recordings showed that of the neurons studied in this experiment, 50% discharged only during movements relative to grasping (*motor neurons*), while the other 50% responded significantly to the sight of the objects, both in the condition in which the viewing was followed by grasping and in that in which the monkey merely fixated the object (*visuomotor neurons*). Two-thirds of the neurons of both types selectively coded a particular prehension modality.

What is most important, however, is that all the visuomotor neurons that showed motor selectivity were also visuo selective. Not only did they discharge more strongly during the fixation of certain geometrical solids as opposed to others, but also the visual selectivity which emerged in condition (C, object fixation) was the same as that found in condition (A) when the monkey was required to grasp the object presented. This was even more surprising as in the (C) condition, differently to (A), the shape of the object was totally irrelevant to the execution of the task, which was to raise the hand from the key. Moreover, a comparison of the selective responses of the visuomotor neurons in the three conditions of the experiment showed that the majority behaved in a similar manner to that illustrated in Figure 2.2, which shows a clear congruency between the motor selectivity of a particular type of prehension and the visual selectivity for objects which, although different in shape and size, have the same prehension coded at motor level.

Similar data have also been reported in humans: fMRI studies[8] have shown that in normal subjects the sight of graspable instruments or objects activates the area of the premotor cortex which is considered to be the human homologue of F5 both when prehension is required and when it is not.

How should these results be interpreted? How is it possible to conciliate the *motor* classification of the F5 neurons with the fact that some of them show *visual* responses at object presentation? How should these responses be interpreted? Could they be the expression of the monkey's intention, of its desire even, to pick up the object? Or should they be attributed to attentional factors? Neither hypothesis is satisfactory, as the neurons should not selectively respond to the objects as was however seen to happen. Intention and attention remain the same, independently of the specific features of the object concerned. Only two possibilities remain: the responses have to be considered either as motor or visual in nature. However, if the motor response is the

---

[8]   See Perani *et al.* (1995); Martin *et al.* (1996); Grafton *et al.* (1997); Chao and Martin (2000); Binkofski *et al.* (1999); Ehrsson *et al.* (2000).

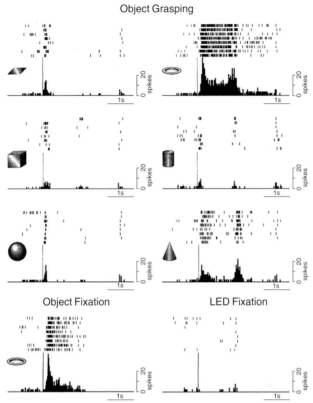

Fig. 2.2 An example of a F5 visuomotor neuron. The upper section of the figure illustrates the activity of the neuron while the monkey observes and grasps various objects. Rasters and histograms are aligned with the instant at which the monkey presses the lever and the object becomes visible. The neuron selectively responds to the ring: of the two response peaks the first is produced by the sight of the ring, the second by the prehension movement. The visual response to the ring is also present in the trials in which the monkey fixates the object without being required to grasp it (lower left panel). Finally, the lower right panel shows the neuron activity when there is no object and the monkey has to fixate a luminous point (Adapted from Murata et al., 1997, 1988.)

correct solution, how are we to explain it in the absence of effective movement?

Before examining these questions that appear to throw doubt on how notions of perception and movement have been traditionally dealt with in neurophysiology, we should continue our analysis of the sensory–motor transformation mechanisms that are involved in acts such as grasping, holding, tearing, etc. It must be remembered that from an anatomical point of view area F5 is closely and mutually connected with the anterior intraparietal area (AIP), whose neurons discharge during hand movements.

Hideo Sataka and his colleagues[9], using an experimental paradigm similar to that subsequently adopted for the study of F5 neurons, showed that on the basis of the responses recorded in the three conditions—(A) grasping in the light; (B) grasping in the dark; and (C) object fixation—it is possible to subdivide the AIP neurons into three categories: *motor dominant*, *visual and motor* and *visual dominant*. The properties of the first two are similar to those of the F5 motor and visuomotor neurons: motor dominant neurons discharge in conditions (A) and (B) but are silent in condition (C); visual and motor neurons are more active in condition (A) than in condition (B), and discharge also in condition (C). The visual dominant neurons, on the other hand, which are not present in F5, discharge in conditions (A) and (C), but not in (B).

Murata *et al.*[10] replicated Sakata's experiment to investigate the visual selectivity of the AIP neurons which are active in conditions (A), (B), and (C) for three-dimensional objects of different geometrical shapes, sizes, and orientation.

---

[9]   Sakata *et al.* (1995).
[10]   Murata *et al.* (2000).

They found that almost 70% of the recorded neurons responded selectively to visual stimuli, and that a fair number of these prevalently code one sole object or a limited number of objects (Figure 2.3).

The functional properties of the neurons would indicate that the AIP–F5 circuit is involved in the visuo-motor transformations which are necessary to grasp an object.

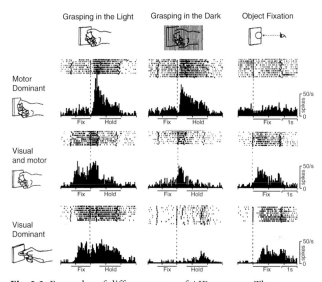

Fig. 2.3 Examples of different types of AIP neurons. The experimental paradigms in the conditions of grasping in the light and object fixation were the same as those for grasping and fixation only in Fig. 2.2. In the grasping in the dark condition, there was a preliminary trial in which the monkey could see the object inside an illuminated box; the light was then switched off and all the successive trials were carried out in the dark. The objects were presented in blocks. The individual trials and the response histograms are aligned with the "go" signal in the grasping conditions and with the start of the task in the fixation condition. (Adapted from Murata et al., 2000.)

However the presence of other hand movement representations in the agranular frontal cortex raises the possibility that the role of this circuit is not as crucial as might be thought. This led to studies on the effects of reversible inactivation of parts of the F5 and AIP areas, produced by microinjections of muscimol which enforces the action of gamma-aminobutyric acid (GABA), one of the most widespread inhibitory neurotransmitters in the central nervous system.

Following the inactivation of AIP, monkeys trained to grasp geometrical solids of varying shapes, sizes, and orientation had great difficulty in shaping the hand contralateral to the damaged hemisphere to the intrinsic characteristics of the objects to be grasped, especially if a precision grip was required. They did occasionally manage to complete the task, but only after repeated corrections to their finger movements based on tactile exploration of the surface of the object.[11]

Inactivation of a portion of F5 produced similar results. However, in this case there was also an evident deficit in the preshaping of the ipsilateral hand though this did not cause any motor impairment (Figure 2.4). This not only shows that F5 exerts bilateral control over hand movements but also that visuo-motor transformation deficits following temporary inactivation of the area are not due to a purely motor impairment.[12]

The hypothesis that visuo-motor transformations connected to grasping depend principally on the AIP–F5 circuit appears to be confirmed by a number of research

---

[11]   See Gallese *et al.* (1994).
[12]   See Fogassi *et al.* (2001).

Grasping
before muscimol injection

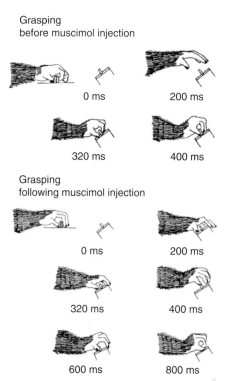

0 ms

200 ms

320 ms

400 ms

Grasping
following muscimol injection

0 ms

200 ms

320 ms

400 ms

600 ms

800 ms

Fig. 2.4 Drawings from videos filmed before and after the temporary activation of a portion of F5 and relative to the hand shaping phases and the grasping of a small object. In this experimental paradigm the monkey was seated in front of a box containing a number of objects differing in size and shape; the side of the box turned towards the monkey was in LCD material. Each trial started when the animal pressed a lever. After 200 msecs, the side of the box facing the monkey became transparent, so that the animal could see the contents. After an interval of time (1.2–1.8 secs.) the side of the box was lowered so that the monkey could reach in and grasp the objects. The time shown under each drawing is calculated from the instant in which the hand started to move. (Adapted from Fogassi et al., 2001.)

studies which have shown that human patients present significant deficits in hand shaping following lesions to the anterior part of the lateral bank of the intraparietal sulcus.[13] This is the same area that, in healthy subjects, is activated by object prehension or manipulation.[14]

The grasping circuit

Just how exactly do AIP and F5 interact? What role do their neurons play in the transformation of visual information into the motor format required for the execution of an act?

We know that one of the most important properties of the visual dominant and visual and motor AIP neurons is that they respond selectively to specific three-dimensional stimuli. Some respond to spherical objects, others to cubes, others again to flat objects, etc. The notion of *affordance*, introduced years ago by James J. Gibson[15], clarifies the functional significance of these responses; it is well known that Gibson held the view that the visual perception of an object implies the immediate and automatic selection of those of its intrinsic properties that facilitate our interaction with it. These are 'not only abstract physical [or geometrical] properties', they incarnate the *practical opportunities* that the object *offers* to the organism which perceives it.[16] Going back to our cup of coffee, the visual affordances offered to our motor system in this case regard the handle, the body of the cup, the brim, etc. As soon as we see the cup, these affordances selectively activate groups of AIP neurons. The visual information is then transmitted to the F5

---

[13] Binkofski *et al.* (1998).
[14] Binkofski *et al.* (1999).
[15] Gibson (1979).
[16] Ibidem, p. 206.

visuomotor neurons which however no longer code the individual *affordances*, but the *motor acts* which are congruent to them. In this way the visual information is translated into motor information and in this format, is sent to area F1 and to the various subcortical centres for the execution of the action.

At present, there are no experimental data that explain how motor responses leading to efficient prehensions, manipulations, etc., gradually came to match the visual aspects of objects. However it is probable that from a very early age we associate certain features of objects with the motor acts that enable us to interact most effectively with them. It is true that the visual information that reaches F5 may seem somewhat disparate; but in time, through feedback circuits, only those which permit us to form adequate motor behaviour will remain. Once we have discovered how to conjugate the different kinds of motor acts with specific visual aspects relative to objects, which therefore become object affordances, our motor system will be able to perform all the transformations necessary to carry out any act, including that of picking up our cup of coffee.

One point still remains to be clarified, however. Many objects, including our coffee cup, have more than one affordance. It follows that when we see these objects, more than one set of neural AIP populations will be triggered, each of which will code a specific *affordance*. It is likely that these *action proposals* will be sent to F5, sparking off what can be defined as *potential motor acts*. Now, the choice of how to act will not depend only on the intrinsic properties of the object in question (its shape, size, and orientation), but also on what we intend to do with it, on its functions, etc. Going back to our coffee cup once more, we will grasp it in different ways depending on whether we are picking it up to drink from it, to rinse it, or simply to move it from one place to another. Moreover, our grip on the cup varies according to the circumstances, whether we are afraid of burning our fingers, or the cup is surrounded by other objects; it will also be influenced by our customs, habits, and our inclination to adhere to certain social rules and so on.

The analysis of the cortical mechanisms underpinning acts such as grasping must take into consideration the processes which underlie the elaboration of this type of information, which would appear to be more motivational or decisional in nature and which involve other areas in the prefrontal lobe, the inferior temporal lobe (IT), and the cingulate cortex, together with the AIP–F5 circuit. In particular, it is thought that the frontal lobe and the areas of the cingulate cortex play a significant role in the decision as to which type of prehension to use, depending on what has to be done and why (for example, whether the cup has to be grasped in order to drink from it or to move it).

There are two lines of thought regarding where this decision actually takes place. According to some authors, it occurs in F5.[17] In this area the appropriate motor act would be selected from a number of potential motor acts indicated by the information supplied by the AIP (Figure 2.5). However, other authors have pointed out that the direct connections between the frontal lobe and F5 are somewhat weak[18], while for some time now it has been accepted that there is a strong connection between the prefrontal cortex and the inferior parietal lobe, including the AIP.[19] It may be, therefore, that the decision is not made in F5 after all, but in

[17]   See, for example, Fagg and Arbib (1998).
[18]   See, for example, Rizzolatti and Luppino (2001).
[19]   Petrides and Pandya(1984).

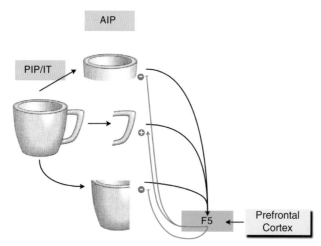

Fig. 2.5 Schematic representation of the AIP-F5 interactions that take place when an individual grasps a cup of coffee. AIP: anterior intraparietal area; IT: inferotemporal cortex; PIP: posterior parietal areas connected with the AIP. The illustration shows that the AIP extracts the visual affordances from objects on the basis of their physical aspect (visual information which comes from the PIP) and their meaning (information supplied by IT) and activates potential motor acts (prehension acts) in F5. On the basis of the intentions of the agent (information supplied by the prefrontal cortex), F5 selects a motor act (in this specific case, a precision grip of the handle) and communicates this choice to the AIP, giving emphasis to the appropriate affordance (the red line ending with +) and suppressing the other affordances (the red lines ending with a −). The transformation of the potential motor act (coded in F5) into an executed act requires the intervention of the mesial cortical areas.

the AIP, and regards the *affordances* and not the motor acts. In other words, on the strength of the information received about a single affordance, F5 decides which is the most appropriate motor act.

The motivational choice is supplemented and integrated by our recognition of the object. For example, a pencil and a pointer have similar affordances, but we hold a pencil (when we need to write with it) in a different way to that in which we hold a pointer. This implies that we recognize the pencil as such and that we can distinguish it from a pointer. As we will see later, the codification of the properties necessary for the recognition of objects takes place in the inferior temporal lobe. It is therefore very likely that the information sent out by this lobe to the AIP is a further factor, over and above the motivational aspect, to be taken into consideration in the choice of the appropriate grip to be used.

The visual streams

The concept that the posterior parietal cortex plays a crucial role in the sensory–motor transformations essential for the execution of visually guided actions is a fundamental assumption that appears also in the model of two visual systems proposed at the beginning of the 1990s by Melvyn Goodale and David Milner.[20]

Ten years earlier, Leslie Ungerleider and Mortimer Mishkin[21] had already proposed a model of two visual systems on the basis of seminal insights on visual organization put

---

[20] Goodale and Milner (1992).
[21] Ungerleider and Mishkin (1982).

forward by David Ingle[22], Colwyn B. Trevarthen[23], and Gerald E. Schneider[24] and above all based on new data that they themselves had obtained from brain lesions in monkeys. They sustained that there are two streams which convey information from the primary visual cortex (area 17 or V1) to the higher centres (Figure 2.6 and the illustration in Figure 2.7). The first, which is in a dorsal position (the *dorsal stream*), terminates in the parietal lobe and is responsible for locating objects. This stream is also known as the *where stream*. The second, which is in a ventral position (the *ventral stream*), terminates in the temporal lobe and mediates the recognition of the figural aspects of objects. It is also known as the *what stream*.

Milner and Goodale[25] accepted the idea that the visual system consists of two functionally different streams, but they suggested that their function is different to that previously proposed. Through a series of ingenious experiments on a patient (DF) who had suffered vast lesions to the occipito-temporal lobe, they showed that DF had relatively normal sight with regard to the elementary visual properties (e.g. visual acuity), but was totally unable to distinguish between even the most basic geometric forms.

The interesting aspect of this case was that although DF's capacity to discriminate forms was badly impaired, she was still able to interact with objects. She was perfectly able to pick up everyday articles—for example, she could catch a ball and even a stick—although the act of grasping a stick requires the extrapolation of highly complex motor dynamics.

---

[22]   Ingle (1967; 1973).

[23]   Trevarthen (1968).

[24]   Schneider (1969).

[25]   Milner and Goodale (1995).

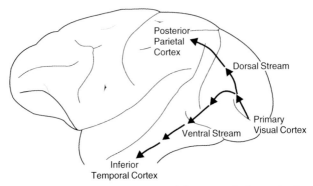

Fig. 2.6 Schematic representation of the anatomical organization of the two visual streams according to the model proposed by Leslie Ungerleider and Mortimer Mishkin. The ventral stream (the *what* stream) is centred in V4 and connects V1 to the inferior temporal cortex (IT) while the dorsal stream (the *where* stream) is centred in the medio-temporal area (MT) and connects the primary visual area (V1) with the areas of the posterior parietal cortex. The model proposed by David Milner and Melvyn Goodale is in accord with that of Ungerleider and Mishkin as far as the ventral stream is concerned, but considers the dorsal stream to be responsible for the *how* of visual information (i.e. information which serves to control actions) and not for the where (space perception).

On the strength of these observations and data obtained from healthy subjects who were able, in certain experimental conditions, to act without being aware of their actions, Milner and Goodale suggested that the fundamental difference between the two streams is not, as Ungerleider and Mishkin thought, in the type of percept (*space* versus *object*) the visual information processing leads to, but the use made of this information by the upper centres. The ventral stream conveys the information necessary to perceive the stimuli and the dorsal stream the information needed to

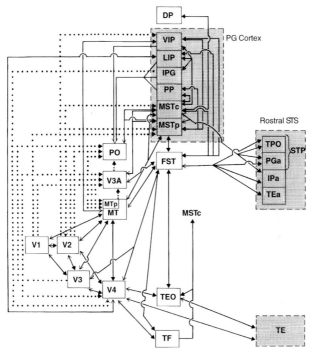

Fig. 2.7 Diagram indicating in detail the visual areas of the two streams (Adapted from Ungerleider, Mishkin, 1982).

control the action. Marc Jeannerod[26] formulated a similar theory in the same period, suggesting that information processing can be either 'semantic' or 'pragmatic'. The former peculiar to the ventral stream, leads to the conscious understanding of the external world, while the latter, typical of the dorsal stream, is dedicated to motor programming.

[26] Jeannerod (1994). For a more sophisticated version of this model see Jacob and Jeannerod (2003) and also Jeannerod (2006).

While credit is undoubtedly due to Goodale and Milner for having demolished the monolithic concept of the visual cortex by attributing it with a role in both motor and perceptive functions, their dichotomic proposal is too rigid to account both for the functional complexities of the parietal lobe and for the clinical pattern which results as a consequence of the lesion. It must also be said that its central assumption, i.e. that perception and action are distinctly separate, reduces the former to a mere iconic representation of the visual properties of objects and relegates the latter to the on-line control processes of the sensory–motor transformations.[27]

The Goodale–Milner model is particularly weak with regard to neglect, the neurological syndrome which typically appears when the right inferior parietal lobule is damaged. Patients suffering from neglect are not able to perceive stimuli arriving from the contralateral space.[28] If for example the experimenter talks to them from their right hand side, they reply as they would normally, but if the experimenter moves to their left hand side and speaks to them, they either ignore him/her, or look for the source of the voice on their right. They ignore food on the left side of their plate, and if they are asked to copy a picture, they copy only the right side and completely ignore the left. In a nutshell, patients suffering from neglect 'lose' the space contralateral to the lesion, or, as Ennio De Renzi put it, their space is 'truncated.[29] It is therefore clear that the dorsal stream does not limit its sphere of activity to controlling movement; it is also involved in perceptive

---

[27] A critical review of the Goodale-Milner model is to be found in Gallese *et al.* (1999).
[28] Bisiach and Vallar (2000).
[29] De Renzi (1982).

processes connected, for example, to the representation of space (see Chapter 3).

These clinical considerations must be integrated with anatomical data. We have already mentioned the high degree of anatomic parcellation of both the superior (SPL) and inferior (IPL) parietal lobules and the importance of the analyses of the frontal parietal connections in understanding the anatomical and functional architecture of the motor system. If we now consider the circuits which process and convey visual information, we can see that the dorsal stream has a much more complex articulation than that which was attributed to it by the Ungerleider–Mishkin and Goodale–Milner models. Recently acquired anatomical and functional knowledge suggests that this stream could well be further divided into two distinct sub-streams: a *ventro-dorsal stream* and a *dorso-dorsal stream*. (Figure 2.8).

The processing and distribution centre of the ventro-dorsal stream is the MT/V5 area, which, as we have seen earlier, is considered to be the node of the dorsal visual system, while the analogous centre for the dorso-dorsal stream is found in V6 (Figure 2.9). MT/V5 and V6 have functional characteristics in common which justify their allocation to the dorsal stream.[30] However, their output does differ significantly: while MT/V5 projects mainly to the areas in the inferior parietal lobule (IPL), V6 is the main source of information for the superior parietal lobule (SPL). Moreover, recent experiments have shown that the IPL has vast access to visual information, predominantly concerning space and biological movements, coded

---

[30]   See Galletti *et al.* (1999; 2001); Gamberoni *et al.* (2002).

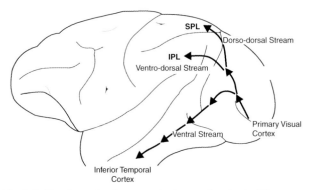

Fig. 2.8 The three visual streams in the monkey brain. The ventral stream is the same as that of the preceding models (see Fig. 2.6), but the dorsal stream is subdivided into a ventro-dorsal stream that terminates in the inferior parietal lobule (IPL) and in a dorso-dorsal stream that terminates in the superior parietal lobule (SPL).

in the superior temporal sulcus (STS) and in particular in the region known as the superior polysensorial temporal area (STP), which is not the case for SPL.[31]

Therefore the dorsal stream as a whole cannot be allocated within the framework of a single functional categorization; we have seen that the dorso-dorsal stream appears to be exclusively, or almost exclusively, involved in the organization of the motor activities through the on-line control features suggested by Milner–Goodale, while the ventro-dorsal stream and the inferior parietal lobule have a variety of motor-perceptive functions which do far more than merely control actions and which overcome any simple dichotomy—independently of whether it concerns the

---

[31] See Rizzolatti and Matelli (2003).

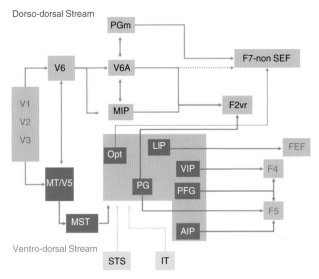

Fig. 2.9 Diagram indicating the anatomical connections of the two dorsal streams. Upper part: dorso-dorsal stream (grey boxes); lower part: ventro-dorsal stream (green boxes). The ventro-dorsal stream receives afferents from areas (yellow boxes) located inside the superior temporal sulcus (STS) and in the inferotemporal lobe (IT)

nature of the percepts (*object* versus *space*, as proposed by Ungerleider and Mishkin) or to how information is used (*vision for perception* versus *vision for action*, as in the Goodale–Milner model).

The vocabulary of acts

In the following chapters we will examine in greater depth the various sensory–motor interaction mechanisms and the interconnection between perception and action. Now, however, we must return to the issues we left open in our analysis of the properties of the F5 neurons and the anterior intraparietal area (i.e. the AIP) as they have become particularly salient in the light of the considerations made on the anatomical and functional organization of the so-called dorsal stream.

As we have already seen, the most surprising aspect that emerged from the single F5 neuron recordings is their selectivity for specific motor acts (grasping, holding, tearing, etc.) and within these acts, for particular execution modalities and activation times. This has led to the hypothesis that F5 contains a form of *vocabulary* of motor acts, in which the *words* are represented by populations of neurons. Some of these indicate the general goal of the act (holding, grasping, breaking, etc.), others the manner in which a specific motor act can be performed (precision grip, finger prehension, etc.) and lastly, there is a group that designates the temporal segmentation of the motor act in its elementary movements (opening and closing of the hand).

This interpretation of F5 in terms of a vocabulary of motor acts has important functional implications. First, the concept of neurons which code specific motor acts explains why our everyday interaction with objects is almost always performed in the same manner. Let us go back to our coffee cup; it can be picked up in many ways of which however we only use a limited number. For example, we never use our middle and ring fingers to grasp the handle. This is probably due to learning mechanisms dating back to our childhood and based on the success of the grip ('motor reinforcement'), which results in a selection of the F5 neurons that code efficient motor acts. Second, a vocabulary would facilitate the association of these acts and the visual affordances extracted by the AIP neurons. Finally, it offers the motor system a 'repertoire' of acts that is at the basis of the cognitive functions that are traditionally attributed to the sensory systems. This will be further discussed in the following chapters.

What we have just described above refers to the motor properties of the F5 neurons. However, we know that a certain percentage of these neurons discharges both during the actual execution of the act *and* while the object is being observed, showing a high level of congruence between the selectivity of the motor responses (the type of grip) and that of the visual responses (the shape, size, and orientation of the object). Responses recorded in the condition in which the object is only observed and no motor act is involved, are immediate, constant, and specific; this would lead us to interpret them as purely visual. However, the same neurons that discharge in those circumstances also become active when the action is to be executed in the light or in the dark, which would justify them being classified as 'motor' neurons.

The only possible interpretation of the behaviour of these neurons is that both visual and motor responses have the same functional meaning. In other words, the messages sent by the F5 visuo-motor neurons to the other centres are exactly the same when the monkey interacts with a certain object (food or geometrical solids) as when the animal merely observes it. When an act is performed, the discharge of the neuron represents the activation of a motor command, such as 'pick this up with a precision grip', but what happens when there is no action involved, just observation? If the neuron also discharges in the same way in this condition, this discharge should convey an identical message to that sent when the animal moves, but which, instead of determining an overt action, remains at the *potential stage*. This happens automatically whenever the monkey looks at a given type of object. If an actual act is required, other areas must be brought into function, such as F6 which receives strong afferents from the prefrontal lobe and is able to modulate motor behaviour. However we must not let our attention be diverted to the control or execution mechanisms; we are interested here in the functions to be ascribed to the vocabulary of motor acts even when there is no explicit intention to act.

The evocation of a potential motor act like grasping is not, in fact, characterized by the specification of the parameters necessary for the execution of the various movements. What it actually does involve is a reference to a particular type of object, characterized by its visuo-motor possibilities.[32]

Once again, our faithful cup of coffee provides an excellent example: the elaboration of the sensory information relative to the shape, size, and orientation of its handle, brim, and so on, is necessary for the process of selection of the type of grip, suggesting a series of movements (starting from those necessary to shape the hand) that enables us to pick up the cup. Whether we succeed or fail in our intent depends on numerous factors such as our ability to execute and control the individual motor processes involved, but this does not change the fact that the cup functions in both cases as a *virtual pole of action*, which, given its relational nature, both defines and is defined by the motor pattern that it activates.

---

[32]   See Livet (1997).

The finding that visuo-motor F5 and AIP neurons respond to object presentation both in executive (grasping an object) and in observation (fixating the same object without picking it up) tasks indicate that the object in question is coded in the same way in both conditions. In other words, the sight of the cup is just a preliminary form of action, a call to arms so to speak, which regardless of whether we actually pick it up, characterizes it as something to be grasped by the handle, with two fingers, etc. and so identifies it in function of the motor opportunities it encompasses.

Returning to the model described in the previous pages, this means that the selection of the visual affordances made in the AIP and the resulting activation in F5 of the congruent potential motor acts are not only at the basis of the commands to the executive areas of the motor system, but they also establish a correlation between the type of prehension and the type of objects that have been coded. If this correlation is successful, the connections built by the AIP–F5 circuit will not only facilitate the activation of the appropriate responses to the visual stimuli but will also categorize objects in terms of possible actions.

It is worth noting that it is very likely that this type of categorization plays a crucial role in the object categorization that infants make in their first months of life. Before semantically recognizing the objects, they categorize them in *small* or *large*, *tilted* or *horizontal*, etc., according to the motor possibilities offered. It is also probable that this motor categorization constitutes the scaffold on which the late visual experience will be constructed, thus providing the source for object semantics.[33]

---

[33]   See Rizzolatti and Gallese (1997).

Seeing with the hand

'We look because we handle, and we are able to handle because we look', are the words used almost a century ago by George Herbert Mead to emphasize how perception would not be possible 'without a continued control of such an organ as that of vision by such an organ as that of the hand, and *vice versa*'.[34] Without this mutual control we would not be able to pick up our cup of coffee. However the analysis of the visuo-motor transformations operated by the AIP–F5 neurons indicates that the seeing which guides the hand is also (and above all) seeing with the hand, by which the object is immediately coded as a given set of invitations to act.[35] The congruence between the visual and motor selectivity of the AIP–F5 neurons shows in fact how, regardless of the parameters which will regulate the actual execution of the act and independently of the latter, their evoked potential motor acts categorize the 'seen' object as *graspable in this* or *that manner*, with *this or that grip*, etc., endowing it with a 'meaning' that it otherwise would not have had.[36] In other words, these neurons appear to respond to the meaning the stimulus conveys to the individual, rather than its sensory aspect, and 'reacting to a meaning is precisely what one means by *understanding*'.[37]

There is no doubt that this 'understanding', which is 'pragmatic' in nature, does not in itself determine a semantic representation of the object, on the basis of which it would be identified and recognized as *a cup of coffee* and

---

[34]   Mead (1907, p. 388).
[35]   See Mead (1938, pp. 23–25).
[36]   Gallese (2000, p. 31).
[37]   Petit (1999, p. 239).

not just a *something that can be picked up by hand*.[38] The F5 and AIP neurons respond only to certain aspects of the object (shape, size, orientation, etc.) and therefore their selectivity is important as these aspects are treated as systems of visual affordances and potential motor acts. On the other hand, the neurons which are located in the inferior temporal cortex code profiles, colours, and textures, processing the selected information into images which, once committed to memory, let us recognize the visual aspects of objects.

After these considerations, is it still possible to maintain that the anatomical distinction between the *ventral* and the *dorsal* streams corresponds to a functional distinction between *vision-for-perception* and *vision-for-action*? We do not believe so—at least, not unless *perception* is reduced to an iconic representation of objects, a depiction of a *thing*, and *action* to mere movement control, absolutely divorced from any relation to the *thing* itself.

We by no means wish to refute the contribution of the areas of the inferior temporal cortex (the ventral stream) to the task of classifying objects (i.e. their identification and conceptualization). Our aim is rather to stress that the function of the motor system is not confined to the execution and control of movements, and that even in the case of simple acts such as grasping, the motor vocabulary contained in the AIP–F5 circuit requires continual interaction between perception and action. However 'pragmatic'[39] it may be, this interaction still plays a decisive role in constructing the sense of objects; without it the majority of the so-called 'higher order' cognitive functions could not take place.

---

[38]   See Jeannerod (1994; 1997).
[39]   Jacob and Jeannerod (2003).

The behaviour of F5 and AIP neurons would therefore help us to re-qualify the notion of perception in the direction indicated by Roger Sperry ('perception is basically an implicit preparation to respond'[40]) and to capture at the neurophysiological level the motor dimension of experience which, in the words of Maurice Merleau-Ponty, 'provides us with a way of access to the world and the object [...] which has to be recognized as original and perhaps as *primary*': 'In the action of the hand which is raised towards an object is contained a reference to the object, [...] as that highly specific thing towards which we project ourselves, near which we are, in anticipation, and which we haunt'.[41]

What really counts, regardless of the specific type of hand motor act involved, and what we see from the analyses of sensory–motor transformations, is that whether these motor acts are actually executed or potentially evoked, they always incorporate the 'orientation and prehension activities' and the 'chains of motor intervention' that Jean-Pierre Changeux and Paul Ricoeur debated in their famous 1998 dialogue, as contributing to organize the world into a 'habitable' environment, 'crisscrossed with viable paths and more or less surmountable obstacles'.[42] In fact, as we will see in the following chapters, the constitution of this 'habitable environment' does not only depend on our picking up this or that object (or our intention to do so), it also requires our capacity to move and to orient ourselves in our surrounding space, as well as our ability to understand the actions and intentions of others.

---

[40]   Sperry (1952).
[41]   Merleau-Ponty (1945, pp. 159, 162).
[42]   Changeux and Ricoeur (1998, p. 137).

CHAPTER 3

The space around us

Reaching for objects

In the preceding chapter, our analysis focussed on the cortical mechanisms which come into play when we grasp our cup of coffee. However, to actually grasp the cup, we have to *reach* it and to do this, we have to *locate* it. In other words, we have to assess its distance from those parts of our body which will be involved in the movement—in the case of our coffee cup, the arm. The act of directing the arm towards the cup requires the brain to undertake a series of processes ranging from coding the spatial relations between the limb and the cup to the transformation of this information into the appropriate motor commands. As in the act of grasping, these processes presuppose specific cortico-cortical interactions between certain areas of the posterior parietal lobe and the agranular frontal cortex.

In the first chapter we have seen that the ventral premotor cortex is formed by area F5 and also by area F4, which lies in its caudal-dorsal portion and receives strong afferents from the inferior parietal lobule, particularly from the ventral intraparietal area (VIP). Experiments using electrical intra-cortical microstimulation have shown that neck, mouth, and arm movements are represented in F4, with the arm movements being directed both towards the body itself and to certain positions in space.[1] Moreover, recordings of single neurons indicate that the majority of F4 neurons become active both during the execution of motor acts and in response to sensory stimuli[2]; consequently these neurons have been classified into two groups: 'somatosensory' neurons and 'somatosensory and visual' neurons, known also as *bimodal* neurons.[3] Recently *trimodal* neurons, which respond to somatosensory, visual, and auditory stimuli, have been recorded.[4]

Most of the F4 *somatosensory* neurons are activated by superficial tactile stimuli: a caress or the sensation of something brushing against the skin is all that is needed to trigger them. Their somatosensory receptive fields are located on the face, neck, arms, and hands; these fields are fairly extensive, covering areas which extend over a number of square centimetres.

The somatosensory characteristics of the *bimodal* neurons are similar to those of the pure somatosensory neurons, but they are triggered also by visual stimuli, particularly three-dimensional objects. Most are susceptible to moving objects (especially objects that are moving in towards the body) although some neurons do respond strongly to stationary objects.[5] Besides these properties, the most interesting functional aspect of F4 bimodal neurons is that they respond to visual stimuli *only* when these appear in the vicinity of their tactile receptive field; more precisely, within that specific space portion which represents their *visual receptive field*

---

[1] Gentilucci *et al.* (1988); Godschalk *et al.* (1984).
[2] Rizzolatti *et al.* (1981 a, b).
[3] Fogassi *et al.* (1992; 1996 a, b); Graziano *et al.* (1994).
[4] Graziano *et al.* (1999).
[5] Fogassi *et al.* (1996 a); Graziano *et al.* (1997).

and appears to constitute an extension of their *somatosensory receptive field*.

Figure 3.1 shows the bimodal receptive fields of some F4 neurons. It should be noted that the visual receptive fields are always located around their respective somatosensory receptive fields. The shape and size of these fields differ, with a depth ranging from just a few centimetres to 40–50 cm. For this reason, the same neuron that discharges when we brush the monkey's forearm also becomes active when we move our hand close to the animal's forearm, entering its visual receptive field. If you find this hard to believe, bring your hand close to your cheek: you will feel it before your fingers actually touch the skin. It is almost as if the personal (i.e. cutaneous) space of your cheek reaches out to embrace the visual space that surrounds it.

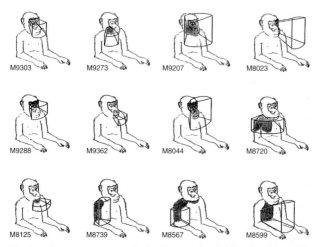

Fig. 3.1 Somatosensory and visual receptive fields of F4 bimodal neurons. The shaded areas indicate the somatosensory receptive fields; the solid figures delineate the visual receptive fields. (Adapted from Fogassi et al., 1996a.)

In this case visual and somatic stimuli are more than just 'equivalent'. As Alain Berthoz stated: '[Spatial-visual] [P]roximity is a form of anticipated contact with the area of the body that will be touched'.[6] The body uses this form of 'anticipated contact' to define its surrounding space, locating its organs (arm, mouth, neck, etc.) and the objects that are in their visual proximity, regardless of whether they are stationary or mobile.

The body's co-ordinates

The most surprising discovery made regarding F4 is that the visual receptive fields of most of the bimodal neurons remain anchored to their respective somatosensory fields and are therefore independent of the direction of the gaze.[7]

This can be best explained with the schematic representation of an experiment (Figure 3.2) illustrating the properties of the visual receptive field of an F4 bimodal neuron and its connection with the somatosensory field. In condition (A1) the monkey is fixating a point (indicated by an asterisk) directly in front of it, while at the same time a visual stimulus (the black arrow) enters its visual receptive field (the stippled area) at a constant speed. The histogram depicting the neuron discharge timing and modalities clearly shows that activation starts when the stimulus is at a distance of approximately 40 cm from the animal. In condition (B1), the monkey's gaze is still directed to the point in front of it, but the stimulus moves to the left of the fixation point, outside the visual receptive field. In this case the neuron does not become active.

---

[6]   Berthoz (1997, p. 69).
[7]   Gentilucci et al. (1983); Fogassi et al. (1996a, b).

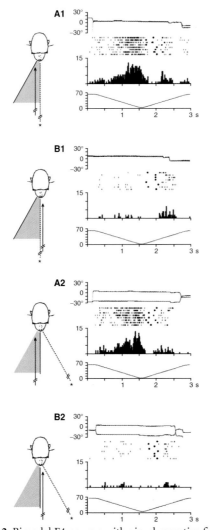

Fig. 3.2 Bimodal F4 neuron with visual receptive field anchored to the body. From top to bottom, the diagrams show the horizontal and vertical eye movements, the neural discharge during individual trials, the response histogram (abscissa: time; ordinate: spikes/bin, bin dimension 20 ms) and the variation over time in the distance between the stimulus and the monkey's head. The descending section of the curve indicates the movement of the stimulus towards the monkey, while the ascending section represents the movement of the stimulus in the opposite direction (abscissa: time in seconds; ordinate: distance in centimetres). The tactile receptive field is localised in the right hemiface. The visual receptive field is positioned around the tactile field. (Adapted from Fogassi et al., 1996a.)

In (A2) the monkey's gaze is moved 30 degrees to the left. Surprisingly enough, although the trajectory followed by the stimulus in this case is totally different in terms of retinal coordinates, the neuron responds in practically the same manner as recorded in (A1). In the last condition(B2) the monkey continues to fixate the same point as (A2), but the stimulus is moved to the right of the fixation point. If the receptive field were coded in retinal coordinates, the response of the neuron should be similar to that in (A1), but in fact the histogram shows that the neuron does not become active.

Overall, this experiment shows that the location of the neuron's visual receptive field does not depend on the position of the stimulus on the retina. If this were the case, when the monkey moved its gaze the visual receptive field should also have shifted, but the experiment shows that this is not so. Numerous experiments have been carried out on F4 bimodal neurons. They show that in 70% of these neurons, their visual receptive fields are linked to their somatosensory fields, coding spatial stimuli in somatic, as opposed to retinal, coordinates.

It is worth remembering at this point that in spite of the position sustained by a number of movement theorists, these coordinates do not refer to a single reference system situated in a specific part of the body such as the head or the shoulders. The fact that the visual receptive fields of F4 bimodal neurons are localized around the somatosensory receptive fields indicates that visual space is coded by a manifold of different body reference systems distributed according to their corresponding somatosensory field. So we have coordinate systems centred on the head, neck, arms, hands, etc., which, as they are anchored to the sensory receptive fields from which they originate, contribute to

locating the visual stimuli in the space surrounding the
body parts to which they are linked.

Imagine just for a minute that you are the mannequin in
Figure 3.3 and that you are fixating the dot on the keyboard
(Figure 3.3A). If you raise your eyes to the computer screen
in front of you (Figure 3.3B), the visual receptive field
(bordered in yellow) anchored to the somatosensory receptive field (the grey shapes) around your mouth and forearm
remain in the same position as before. Now, if you turn to
look at the cup of coffee on your right and move to pick it
up (Figure 3.3C), the pericutaneous visual receptive fields
move. This does not depend on the direction of your gaze,

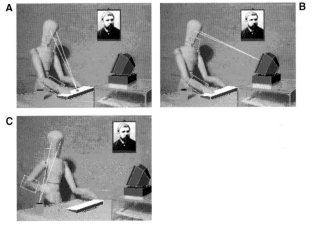

Fig. 3.3 This set of three drawings illustrates the independence of
the F4 visual receptive fields with respect to the direction of the
gaze. A detailed explanation is given in the text. The portrait of
Jules-Henri Poincaré will not have escaped the attention of the
attentive reader; we are convinced that the French mathematician
would have appreciated this experiment and its results. (Adapted
from Rizzolatti et al., 1997.)

but on the position of your head and forearm, or, in other words, on the position of the somatosensory receptive fields.

For the sake of simplicity we have described just two of the many receptive fields present in the body and only one form of movement (rotation of the trunk and the head). But our mannequin, like the monkeys shown in Figure 3.1, possesses many peripersonal receptive fields, some of which cover cup location. But what happens when our mannequin moves its hand towards the cup? Irrespective of the direction of its gaze, the position of the cup with respect to its hand, forearm, etc. is specified by the appropriate pericutaneous visual receptive fields. Their stimulation anticipates the actual contact with the skin, so that its hand does not have to physically touch the cup to 'know' where it is; it is sufficient for the hand to be close enough to trigger the neurons through its visual receptive fields. As these fields are simply a three-dimensional extension of the respective cutaneous fields, the visual individuation of that cup should initiate the specific movements of the arm which propel the hand towards it just as if it were a tactile stimulus, without any need to convert the visual coordinates into any other form (which would be extremely complex and onerous).

Near and far

The presence of visual receptive fields in F4 and the VIP which is closely connected to it [8], not only throws light on the sensory–motor transformations suggested by the acts of locating and reaching for an object, it also throws doubt

---

[8] Similar receptive fields have also been found in the PF area which is situated in the convexity of the inferior parietal lobe. For further details, see Fogassi *et al.* (1996); Rizzolatti *et al.* (2000) among others.

on the traditional concept of a single spatial map. This concept in fact hypothesized a single spatial map located in the parietal lobe to be used for multiple purposes (e.g. eye, head, trunk and arm movements, etc.). [9] In the first chapter we wrote at length on the anatomical parcellation of the parietal cortex, by which it is organized into a series of circuits that operate in parallel. This anatomical organization is totally incompatible with the concept of a unitary cortical representation of space. If we go on to consider the functional properties of the various areas which constitute the parietal lobe and process spatial information through their connections with the occipital and frontal lobes, it is evident that they operate in a completely different manner. This is due to the fact that they control different motor goals and have their own visual input.

When the functional properties of the VIP–F4 circuit are compared to that formed by the lateral intraparietal area (LIP) and the frontal eye fields (FEF), the difference becomes very clear. The role of the latter circuit is to control the rapid eye movements (also known as *saccadici*), whose function is to focus the fovea on targets located in the periphery of the visual field. In both these circuits the neurons respond to visual stimuli and discharge in association with particular types of movement, but the similarities end here. In the LIP–FEF areas, in fact, the neurons respond to the visual stimulus independently of the distance at which this is located; their visual receptive fields are coded in retinal coordinates (i.e. each field has its specific position on the retina relative to the fovea); their motor properties concern eye movements only.[10] On the other hand, as we

---

[9]   For example, see Stein (1992).
[10]   See Andersen *et al.* (1997); Colby and Goldberg (1999).

have already seen, the VIP–F4 neurons are mostly bimodal and respond more strongly to three-dimensional objects than to simple luminous stimuli; their receptive fields are coded in somatic coordinates and anchored to various parts of the body[11]; last but not least, the visual stimuli must appear within the pericutaneous space to activate them. In other words, they must appear in the spatial region which includes all the objects at arm's length and which for convenience sake we will call *peripersonal* or *near space* to distinguish it from the *extrapersonal* or *far space* which is beyond the reach of our limbs.[12]

There are two points here that deserve particular attention: first, that the LIP–FEF and VIP–F4 circuits use different coordinate systems and second, the type of movement they control encompasses the distinction between our peripersonal space and that which is beyond our immediate reach.

Let us take a minute to consider the first point: the neurons that convey spatial information to LIP–FEF have visual receptive fields coded in retinal coordinates that are adequate for programming simple eye movements. If a pinpoint of light appears 5 degrees to the right of our fovea we have to move our eyes 5 degrees to reach it; in other words there is a direct correspondence between the position of the pinpoint of light and the magnitude of the eye movement required. However it is not always so. Take for example another case in which two pinpoints of light are switched on in rapid sequence, while the observer keeps his eyes still. The first is 5 degrees to his right, the other 5 degrees to his left.

---

[11]   Gentilucci et al. (1983; 1988); Graziano and Gross (1995; 1997; 1998).
[12]   Rizzolatti, *et al.* (1983).

He is asked to fixate them one after the other. In this case, the retinal coordinates are not sufficient to complete the task successfully; in fact, they indicate that two movements are required to reach the pinpoints of light, one of 5 degrees to the right and the other of 5 degrees to the left. If the observer were to entrust this task exclusively to the retinal coordinates, he would carry out the first part of the task correctly (moving 5 degrees to the right) but would not be able to reach the second pinpoint, as this requires a movement of 10 degrees which is not signalled by the retina.

With the exception of very basic tasks, the ocular motor system requires a coordinate system that can calculate the position of the objects in the surrounding space as a function of the observer, and not of their position on the retina. A number of models have been proposed to explain how it is possible to pass from a system of retinal coordinates to one that is able to code a position in space. One of the most well-known[13], though not universally accepted, models places great emphasis on a category of neurons in the lateral intraparietal area; these neurons have receptive fields which signal the position of the stimulus on the retina (the retinal coordinates), but whose response to the visual stimuli is modulated by the position of the eye in its orbit (orbital effect). Once the observer knows where the stimulus is on the retina and where the eye is in its orbit, by a computation requiring a large number of neurons he can calculate the location of the object and direct his gaze onto it.[14]

It is clear that the system of coordinates used by the VIP–F4 circuit to locate objects in space is radically different.

---

[13]   Zipser and Andersen (1988).
[14]   Other solutions are to be found in Bruce (1988); Goldberg and Bruce (1990); Goldberg *et al.* (1990) among others.

Here space is coded in somatic coordinates centred on various parts of the body; the specification of the spatial position of the stimulus relative to these coordinates is processed at the *single neuron* level and does not require the combined effort of a multiplicity of neurons. As already mentioned, the visual receptive fields of the bimodal VIP–F4 neurons are anchored to their respective somatosensory receptive fields and therefore to various parts of the body (hands, arms, neck, etc.), so the stimulus is located independently of the position of the eyes. This greatly simplifies the organization of the movements of those body parts, as they consistently offer the best reference system possible.

Studies on deficits following lesions of FEF and F4 in the monkey appear to confirm the functional subdivision of space into *near* and *far*.[15] In FEF lesions, the impairment principally affects extrapersonal space, while lesions of F4 mostly affect peripersonal space and what is known as personal or cutaneous space.

Similar results have been observed in research conducted on humans with spatial neglect. Peter W. Halligan and John C. Marshall described the case of a patient whose neglect was evident when asked to use a pencil to bisect segments drawn on a piece of paper in his peripersonal space. However, when the paper was moved to his extrapersonal space and he was asked to perform this task with a laser pen, the neglect greatly diminished—in fact, it disappeared almost completely. This explains why he was still able to enjoy his favourite hobby: darts![16] Alan Cowey and his co-workers reported the case of five patients with the opposite form of

---

[15]   Rizzolatti *et al.* (1983).
[16]   Halligan and Marshall (1991). See also Berti and Frassinetti (2000); Berti and Rizzolatti (2002).

neglect; the impairment of their extrapersonal space was much more severe than of the peripersonal space.[17]

The neural organizations in humans and monkeys not only have the near/far distinction in common; the peripersonal space of both is coded by a system of bimodal neurons. When testing responses to visual and tactile stimuli in a patient with evident somatosensory extinction (a clinical picture characterized by the fact that when two symmetric stimuli are shown simultaneously, one on the left and one on the right hand side, the patient perceives only the stimulus on the side unaffected by the lesion) Giuseppe di Pellegrino and co-workers[18] discovered that as soon as a visual stimulus was presented *close* to the patient's right hand, on the same side as the lesion, he no longer perceived the tactile stimulus of a light touch to the hand affected by the lesion (i.e. his left hand). What was most interesting of all, however, was that when the visual stimulus was shown *outside* the patient's peripersonal space, the visual extinction effect on his sense of touch was very weak, or absent altogether.

Considering the role played by F4 and VIP in the processing of spatial information in the monkey, it is not unlikely that the phenomena described by di Pellegrino and his colleagues had a substrate of bimodal neurons. It is worth noting here that an fMRI study has localized certain polymodal areas (activated by tactile, visual, and auditory stimuli)[19] in the human brain. In particular a significant polymodal convergence has been found at the floor of the intraparietal sulcus (IP), in the ventral premotor cortex and the cortex

---

[17]   Cowey *et al.* (1994). This form of dissociation was found again by Cowey and reported in Cowey *et al.* (1999); Vuillemieur *et al.* (1998); Frassinetti *et al.* (2001).

[18]   di Pellegrino *et al.* (1997); see also Làdavas *et al.* (1998a).

[19]   Bremmer *et al.* (2001).

around the secondary somatosensorial area (SII). Although it is difficult to draw a conclusion regarding the role of the SII on the basis of the data currently available, the anatomical position and the properties of the IP and the ventral premotor cortex lead us to believe that these are the human homologues of the VIP and F4 areas in the monkey.

Poincaré's duel

Far from taking the form of a unitary map, the cortical representation of space in both humans and monkeys appears to be based on the activation of distinct sensory–motor circuits, each of which organizes and controls motor acts (such as reaching) that require objects to be specifically located with respect to a given body part (hand, mouth, eyes, etc.). However we still have to discuss the nature of this spatial representation and its relation to the visuo-motor responses of the F4 and VIP neurons.

Here we find a similar problem to that discussed in the preceding chapter: as in F5 and AIP, there are neurons in F4 and VIP which discharge both during the animal's active movements and in response to visual stimuli. There is no doubt that the type of coded act is different (grasping and holding in the first case, reaching in the second). Nevertheless, the presence in both neural circuits of visual responses connected to motor activation suggests that what is true for objects is equally true for space. In other words, the discharge of the F4–VIP neurons does not merely indicate the position of the stimulus within a visual space on the basis of a system of coordinates, but elicits a potential motor act directed towards that stimulus, describing its position in terms of possibility of action.

The very fact of the existence of peripersonal space coded in somatic coordinates would appear to lend substance to this interpretation. If we were to consider peripersonal space as being primarily visual, basing this assumption on, for example, the constancy and high fidelity with which F4 neurons respond to the presentation of a stimulus, it would be difficult to provide an explanation as to why eyes with normal refraction and accommodation should select luminous stimuli coming only from the spatial region surrounding the body of the observer — unless of course we were to resort to some form of *ad hoc* hypothesis, assuming, for example, that F4 contains a complicated mechanism which eliminates visual information coming from beyond peripersonal space. The question is, do we really need this mechanism? Would it not be simpler and more economical to posit that the motor properties of these neurons (their 'vocabulary of acts', as explained in the previous chapter), contribute significantly to determining the distinction between *near* and *far*, creating a space for action within what would otherwise be undifferentiated visual information? After all, what is peripersonal space if not what we can reach by stretching out our hands?

When all is said and done, by insisting on the essentially active nature of the representation of coded space at the level of the premotor cortex and the inferior parietal lobe, we are reiterating the lesson of Ernst Mach, the great physician and physiologist (and philosopher, although he tended to avoid defining himself as such). Almost a century ago, he wrote that 'the points of physiological space' are nothing other than the 'goals of various movements of grabbing, looking and locomotion'.[20] These movements are the starting point from which our body *maps* the space that surrounds us, and it is due to their goal-directedness that space acquires form for us.

---

[20]   Mach (1905, p. 260).

This concept was also familiar to another great mathematician and physicist, Jules-Henri Poincaré. Unlike Mach, Poincaré was not averse to being termed a philosopher, but they did have in common years of study spent on the genesis and structure of spatial representation. According to Poincaré, in fact, not only is it necessary to 'discard the idea of a presumed sense of space …'[21], we must also recognize that 'we could not have constructed space if we had not an instrument for measuring it'—an instrument 'to which we refer everything' and 'which we use instinctively', which is *our body*. In Poincaré's words: 'It is in reference to our own body that we locate exterior objects, and the only special relations of these objects that we can picture to ourselves are their relations with our body.'[22]

In Poincaré's view, these 'relations' are to be construed in terms of motor acts, by which we can reach the objects that surround us:

> For instance, at a moment α the presence of an object A is revealed to me by the sense of sight; at another moment β the presence of another object B is revealed by another sense, that, for instance, of hearing or of touch. I judge that this object B occupies the same place as the object A. What does this mean? […] The impressions that have come to us from these objects have followed absolutely different paths [… and] have nothing in common from the qualitative point of view. The representations we can form of these two objects are absolutely heterogeneous and irreducible one to the other. Only I know that, in order to reach the object A, I have only to extend my right arm in a certain way; even though I refrain from doing it, I represent to myself the muscular and other analogous sensations which accompany that extension, and

---

[21]   Poincaré (1913, pp. 97–98).
[22]   Poincaré (1908, p. 100).

that representation is associated with that of the object A. Now I know equally that I can reach the object B by extending my right arm in the same way, an extension accompanied by the same train of muscular sensations. And I mean nothing else but this when I say that these two objects occupy the same position. I know also that I could have reached the object A by another appropriate movement of the left arm, and I represent to myself the muscular sensations that would have accompanied the movement. And by the same movement of the left arm, accompanied by the same sensations, I could equally have reached the object B. And this is very important, since it is in this way that I could defend myself against the dangers with which the object A or the object B might threaten me. With each of the blows that may strike us, nature has associated one or several parries which enable us to protect ourselves against them. The same parry may answer to several blows. It is thus, for instance, that the same movement of the right arm would have enabled us to defend ourselves at the moment α against the object A, and at the moment β against the object B. Similarly, the same blow may be parried in several ways, and we have said, for instance, that we could reach the object A equally well either by a certain movement of the right arm, or by a certain movement of the left. All these parries have nothing in common with one another, except that they enable us to avoid the same blow, and it is that, and nothing but that, we mean when we say that they are movements ending in the same point of the space. Similarly, these objects, of which we say that they occupy the same point in space, have nothing in common, except that the same parry can enable us to defend ourselves against them.[23]

If we substitute 'representation of sensations' with 'potential motor act', and if we keep in mind the 'anticipatory' function with respect to the cutaneous contact guaranteed

---

[23]   Ibidem (pp. 101–102) (italics placet by the authors).

by the three-dimensional extension of F4 receptive fields, it would be hard to find a better description of the region of space that we term 'peripersonal' and Poincaré defined in terms of the mutual 'co-ordination' resulting from 'the multiplicity of [possible] parries.'[24] Taking this further, as these parries involve 'the lowest parts of the nervous system', according to Poincaré the resulting co-ordination would not be a conquest by the 'individual', but by the 'species', and in fact 'traces' of it can already be seen in the newly born infant.

> The more necessary these conquests were, the more quickly they must have been brought about by natural selection. On this account those we have been speaking of must have been among the earliest, since without them the defence of the organism would have been impossible. As soon as the cells were no longer merely in juxtaposition, as soon as they were called upon to give mutual assistance to each other, some such mechanism as we have been describing must necessarily have been organized in order that the assistance should meet the danger without miscarrying.[25]

Taken in the context of evolution, the *near/far* dichotomy as well as the connections between the motor possibilities of the various parts of the body and the codification modalities of the spatial relations lose much of the mystery that surrounded them at first glance. Space would no longer be represented *per se* somewhere in the cerebral cortex; its construction would depend on the activity of the neural circuits whose primary function is to organize movements which, albeit through different effectors (hands, mouth, eyes, etc.), ensure interaction with the surroundings, locating possible threats and opportunities.

---

[24]   Ibidem (p. 104).
[25]   Ibidem (pp. 103–104).

In any case, the hypothesis that space is primarily constituted in terms of potential motor acts becomes clear if we
follow Poincaré's lead and consider the 'traces' already present in new-born babies. Modern-day ultrasound techniques
show that the unborn child engages in various motor activities in the womb: for example, after the eighth week it
moves its hands towards its face, and in the sixth month of
gestation it is able to put its thumb in its mouth to suck it.
This demonstrates that even before birth babies possess
motor representations of space.[26] After birth, their movements are increasingly goal-directed and clearly referred to
the space around their body. The optical condition is
congruent with the motor situation. As the crystalline lens
is not completely operational at that age, the focal distance
is more or less fixed and babies can only see clearly objects
that are within 20 cm. In this way, they acquire a representation of their peripersonal space (directions and depth)
without having to distinguish whether a stimulus is *near*
or *far*. They can therefore use their motor knowledge to
construct space to associate with the arm movement developed in the womb, first when the hand appears in different
spatial positions and later when objects appear in the same
position. Jean Piaget observed that three-month-old children spend much of their time watching their hands[27] and
this is probably to be ascribed to the necessity of calibrating
peripersonal space in addition to that of measuring object
sizes according to their graspability.

Eye movements, especially the capacity to converge the
eyes, develop during the first three months of life, and the
information the new-born derives from this activity, together

---

[26]   See Butterworth and Harris (1994).
[27]   Piaget (1936). See also Berti and Rizzolatti (2002).

with data from hand and head movements, helps children refine their peripersonal space. At three months, when the constitution of this space is complete and the lens has developed, they can look into the distance. Using their knowledge of peripersonal space and correlating visual stimuli from far off with movements of the hand and eyes and of other parts of the body, babies can start constructing their extrapersonal space.

A dynamic concept of space

The motor constitution of space, by which it appears as a system of coordinated actions, provides us with the opportunity of clarifying one aspect of the near/far dichotomy that would be difficult to explain with the exclusively sensory interpretation of spatial representation codified by the various parieto-frontal circuits, including those formed by VIP–F4. Once again Poincaré's words supply an excellent illustration:

> There are points that will always remain out of my reach, whatever effort I may make to stretch out my hand to them. If I were attached to the ground, like a sea-polyp, for instance, which can only extend its tentacles, all these points would be outside space, since the sensations we might experience from the action of bodies placed there would not be associated with the idea of any movement enabling us to reach them, or with any appropriate parry. These sensations would not seem to us to have any spatial character, and we should not attempt to locate them. But we are not fixed to the ground like the inferior animal. If the enemy is too far off, we can advance upon him first and extend our hand when we are near enough. This is still a parry, but a long-distance parry.[28]

---

[28]   Poincaré (1908, p. 105).

The 'parry' as such contributes to establishing the spatial position of objects which previously did not have such a position, as they were *out* of hand's reach. However, as Poincaré reminds us, hand-reach is not fixed, as its space cannot be conceived as *static*, but as *dynamic*. In other words, the distinction between *near* and *far* cannot be reduced to a mere question of centimetres, as it could be if our brain calculated the distance separating the objects in our vicinity from our body in absolute terms. Not only would this concept of rigid and fixed peripersonal space contradict the principle of spatial relativity held by Poincaré and, as we have seen, essential to the body's organization of movement, it is also incompatible with the organization of the F4 visual receptive fields and the anticipatory function they serve with regard to cutaneous contact.

If we turn back to Figure 3.1, we can see that not only do the extensions of the various visual receptive fields differ, but there are several F4 neurons that do not have a clear boundary. However, the most important aspect to note is that for many bimodal neurons *an increase in the speed at which the stimulus approaches expands their receptive fields in depth.*[29] The fact that the depth of the receptive fields augments with the increase of the speed at which the stimulus approaches, often produces an advance warning system; rapidly approaching stimuli are signalled while they are still at a greater distance from the body compared to stimuli approaching more slowly. The advantage is quite obvious; the earlier the neuron discharges, the earlier the motor act it codes is evoked. This advance action leaves more time for an efficient mapping of the space, to reach the opportunity or avoid the threat.

---

[29] Fogassi *et al.* (1996a). See also Chieffi *et al.* (1992).

There is another way that F4 neurons can redefine the space surrounding the codified effectors. Poincaré reminded us to keep locomotion in mind; locomotion, however, involves the displacement of the numerous reference systems anchored to the various parts of the body rather than the effective transformation of peripersonal space. New objects certainly appear within this space, and are located, but the boundaries of *near space* in this condition as such do not appear to change with regard to the body; rather, they move with it. This notwithstanding the example provided by Poincaré contains a valuable indication: unlike the sea-polyp, humans (and non-human primates) can approach objects (or parry threats) wielding an *instrument*.

Atsushi Iriki and co-workers[30] have shown how in monkeys the visual receptive fields of the bimodal neurons of the posterior parietal cortex, which code the movements of the hand in a manner similar to that of F4 neurons, can be modified by actions which involve the use of tools. They trained some monkeys to recuperate pieces of food with a small rake and observed that when the instrument was used repeatedly, the receptive fields anchored to the hand expanded to encompass the space around both the hand and the rake, almost as if the image of the rake were incorporated in that of the hand.[31] If the animal stopped using the rake, but continued to hold it, the receptive fields returned to their normal extension. The use of the rake enlarged the animal's peripersonal space and therefore remodelled the distinction between *near* and *far*: in other words, the neurons that discharged in the presence of

---

[30]   Iriki *et al.* (1996).
[31]   See also Aglioti *et al.* (1996).

objects in the peripersonal space also responded to stimuli which they had not codified previously when they were at a distance (*far*—outside their space), but which, due to the use of the rake, entered the animal's *near* space.

A similar remodelling of spatial maps has been observed in humans. Anna Berti and Francesca Frassinetti[32] have shown how cortical representation of body space can be extended to include instruments used, with the result that space which was previously codified as *far* becomes *near*. Their patient had suffered a severe right hemisphere lesion that had caused left hemineglect with evident dissociation between peripersonal and extrapersonal space. Tasks which required her to perform actions in her peripersonal space such as reading, line cancellation and bisection, revealed severe deficits; for example, when she was asked to indicate the midpoint of a number of slanted lines drawn on a sheet of paper, she always moved it to the right, a clear evidence of the fact that she was suffering from perceptive deficits with regard to the left side of the lines. As soon as the paper was moved a certain distance (approximately one metre) away so that she had to use a laser pen to perform the task, the neglect tended to disappear.

At first glance this case appears to be very similar to that of Halligan and Marshall; however, something new emerged from Berti and Frassinetti's experiment: when the patient was required to bisect lines in her extrapersonal space with a rod which allowed her to *reach* them, the neglect was also apparent in her far space and was just as severe as in her peripersonal space. Just as the use of an instrument had extended the peripersonal space of the monkeys studied by Iriki and colleagues, the use of the rod appeared to extend

---

[32]   Berti and Frassinetti (2000). See also Berti *et al.* (2001).

the peripersonal space of Berti and Frassinetti's patient to the lines that she was required to bisect. Her far space was re-coded as near space, and consequently was affected by neglect: in fact, the use of the rod extended her neglect of her peripersonal space to her extrapersonal space.

The variable reach of our actions

Objects and space seem therefore to refer to a pragmatic constitution by which the former appear as *poles of virtual acts* and the latter is defined by *the system of relations* deployed by these acts and anchored to the various parts of the body. The neural circuits involved are obviously different, just as the typologies of acts that they codify are different.

Nevertheless, however distinct they may be, and although they operate in parallel to each other, these processes are modulated by *action*. We have mentioned several times that the vocabulary of acts located in F5 and F4 does not contain references to individual movements and how the functions of the premotor cortex can only be fully comprehended if it is clearly understood that these areas code goal-centred representations of movement. As we have seen, we do not extend our arm towards an object unless we intend to inter-act with it, to grasp, or maybe just parry it.

Once again, the coffee cup provides a useful example: from the very first movement towards opening the hand, our brain selects those aspects of the cup (shape and orien-tation of the handle, brim, and so on) which appear relevant to the action to be undertaken and which contribute to establishing both the *motor physiognomy* of the cup and the *space of the possible grips*. The former takes its substance from the latter and vice versa. Having said this, for the prehension to be effective the cup has to be *within reach*, and *localizable* for the body parts which will be involved in the act of grasping. The space of the object is now that of its position relative to the various body parts (arm, hand, mouth, and so on) involved in the act and is defined in terms of their possible goal-directed movements. These may vary from time to time, but they are never divorced from the localization of the object in space.

In fact, if that were the case, the space that surrounds us would be nothing more than an undifferentiated set of points. However, we have learned from the preceding analysis, and from the genial insights of Mach and Poincaré, that space takes its form initially from the objects and the numerous coordinated acts that allow us to reach out to them. It follows that objects are simply *hypotheses of action* and therefore places in space cannot be interpreted as 'objective positions' in relation to an equally alleged objective position of the body, but must be understood, as Merleau-Ponty pointed out, in their 'marking, in our vicinity, the varying range of our aims and our gestures'.[33] This range dictates our possibility of distinguishing between peripersonal as opposed to extrapersonal space and of understanding the dynamic nature of the boundary that separates one from the other.

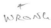

The close connection between objects and space also clarifies a question which is frequently overlooked in studies on spatial neglect, which, as we have observed earlier, concerns some basic aspects of spatial representation (codification of peripersonal space, its possible expansion, etc.). It is important to remember that spatial neglect also prevents perception of objects, as has been shown by various studies.[34] This phenomenon is probably best illustrated by the case

---

[33]   Merleau-Ponty (1945, p. 166).
[34]   See Volpe *et al.* (1979); Berti and Rizzolatti (1992); Marshall and Halligan (1988).

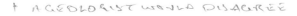

described by Marshall and Halligan[35] in which a patient suffering from a very pronounced left hemineglect was shown two drawings of a house in rapid succession. The right hand side of the house was identical in both drawings, but in one drawing the left side of the house was devoured by flames; the patient declared that she saw no difference, although when asked in which house she would prefer to live she always indicated the drawing without the flames. So, although she was—unconsciously—able to discriminate between the two stimuli, the spatial neglect caused by lesions to the parieto-frontal circuits prevented her *locating* them and *grasping* them, even only by sight.

This is additional confirmation of the interdependence of the constitution of objects and space which emerges from their common action base, and in virtue of which the impossibility of reaching the former goes hand in hand with the impossibility of mapping the various regions of the latter. It underlines the shortcomings of any rigidly dichotomic interpretation of the functioning of our brain, such as those described in the preceding chapter and based on the contraposition of the *what* stream and the *where* stream, or of the *what* stream and the *how* stream. Ranging from the classification of objects to spatial representation, the motor system (in particular the cortical areas located in the *ventro-dorsal stream*) demonstrates a wealth of functions far exceeding the mere control of movement. These functions are connected to action dynamics, which, as we will see in the coming chapters, involve not only our body and the objects that surround it but also the bodies of others in action.

---

[35]   Marshall and Halligan (1988).

CHAPTER 4

Action understanding

Canonical neurons and mirror neurons

From the analysis of the functional properties of F5 we have seen that the majority of neurons in this area discharge during specific motor acts such as grasping, holding, manipulating, and how some of them *also* respond to visual stimuli. There is a clear congruence between the motor properties (for example, the type of grip they code) of these latter neurons and their visual selectivity (shape, size, orientation of the object in question), which renders decisive their role in the process of transforming the visual information regarding an object into the appropriate motor acts. These neurons have been called *canonical neurons*, because for a long time it was thought that the premotor cortex might be involved in visuo-motor transformations.

However, experiments carried out on monkeys in the early 1990s, in which the monkey had not been trained to perform specific tasks but was able to act freely, revealed that these were not the only type of neurons with visuo-motor properties.[1] Surprisingly, neurons were found which became active *both* when the animal itself executed a motor act (for example, when it grasped food) and when it observed the experimenter doing it. These neurons were

---

[1] di Pellegrino *et al.* (1992).

recorded in the cortical convexity of F5 and were named *mirror neurons*.[2]

The *motor properties* of the mirror neurons are identical to those of other F5 neurons in that they discharge selectively during specific motor acts, but their *visual properties* differ significantly. Unlike the canonical neurons, mirror neurons do not discharge at the sight of food or other three-dimensional objects, nor does their behaviour appear to be influenced by the size of the visual stimuli. In fact, their activation depends on the observation of specific motor acts involving a body part (hand or mouth)—object interaction. It is interesting to note that mimed motor acts or intransitive actions (i.e. without a correlated object) such as raising the arms or waving the hands, do not elicit neuron response. Another point worthy of mention is that the discharge of mirror neurons is largely uninfluenced by the distance and spatial location of the observed act in relation to the observer—although in some cases they appear to be affected by the direction of the movements seen or the hand (left or right) used by the experimenter.

If we take the effective motor act, coded *visually*, as the distinguishing criterion, mirror neurons can be subdivided into classes akin to those applied to the motor properties of F5 neurons in Chapter 2: thus we have 'grasping-mirror-neurons', 'holding-mirror-neurons', 'manipulating-mirror-neurons', but also 'placing-mirror-neurons' (which discharge when the monkey sees the experimenter placing an object on a stand) and 'interacting-with-hands-mirror-neurons' (which trigger at the sight of a hand which moves in the direction of the other hand while the latter is holding an object). This classification reveals that most F5 mirror neurons

---

[2] Rizzolatti *et al.* (1996a); Gallese *et al.* (1996).

trigger when a *specific type of act* is observed (grasping, for example). Other neurons do not seem to be so selective, discharging during observation of two, sometimes (but rarely) three, motor acts.

Figure 4.1 illustrates the behaviour of a typical 'grasping-mirror-neuron'. In condition (A), the monkey observes the experimenter while he lifts a piece of food from a tray. The neuron starts to discharge as soon as the experimenter's hand approaches the food and begins to assume the shape required to pick it up; the discharge continues until the act is concluded. In condition (B), the monkey picks up the food and in this case also the discharge of the neuron is correlated to the shaping of the hand.

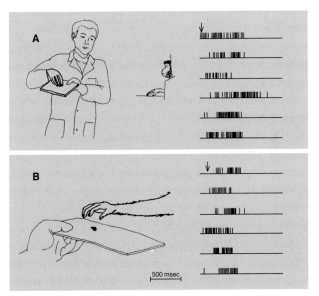

Fig. 4.1 Visual and motor responses of a "grasping-mirror-neuron". (di Pellegrino et al., 1992.)

A comparison of the visual responses and the activity during motor acts reveals one of the most important functional aspects of the mirror neurons: the congruence between the coded motor act and the observed motor act which triggered it.

However, different neurons have different degrees of congruence. Two main types have been identified: *strictly congruent* and *broadly congruent*. In *strictly congruent* neurons the correspondence between the action observed and that executed is virtually exact; an example is provided in Figure 4.2. In condition (A), the monkey observes the experimenter twisting a raisin in his hands, anti-clockwise and clockwise, as if to break it in two: the neuron discharges for one direction only. In condition (B), the experimenter and the monkey both have a grip on the same raisin: the neuron discharges when the animal turns its wrist in the direction opposite to that of the experimenter so as to break the raisin. In condition (C), the monkey picks up the food using a precision grip. This motor act does not produce any discharge.

In *broadly congruent* neurons, the acts coded by the neuron in visual and motor terms are clearly connected, though not identical, and their link can present different levels of generality. In fact some neurons respond to only one performed motor act (grasping, for example) and to two observed acts (grasping and holding). Others code a single executed and observed motor act, but with a different degree of selectivity. Take for example the neuron in Figure 4.3. It discharges when the monkey observes the experimenter grasping an object with a precision grip or with a whole hand prehension, but it responds only when the animal itself uses a precision grip to pick up the object. Then there

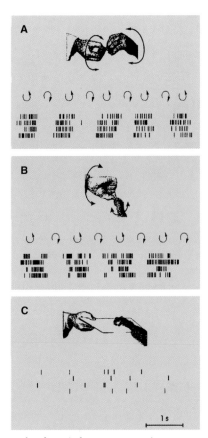

Fig. 4.2 Example of a strictly congruent mirror neuron. A. The monkey observes the experimenter twisting a raisin in his hands with an anti-clockwise and clockwise movement: the neuron becomes active for one direction only. B. The experimenter rotates a piece of food that the monkey is holding in its hand, and animal turns its wrist in the direction opposite to that of the experimenter. C. The monkey picks up the food with a precision grip. Four series of recordings are shown for each experimental condition. The arrows above the discharge recordings indicate the direction of the rotation. (Rizzolatti et al., 1996a.)

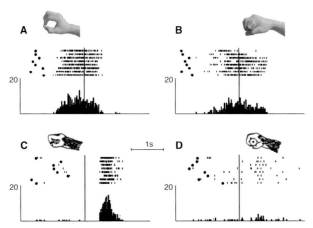

Fig. 4.3 Example of a broadly congruent neuron. A. The experimenter grasps a piece of food with a precision grip. B. The experimenter grasps a piece of food with a whole hand prehension. C. The monkey picks up the food with a precision grip. The neuron is highly selective for active grasping, but not for grasping observation (Adapted from Gallese et al., 1996.)

are neurons which code an action visually, while discharging during the performance of another action which is correlated with the first. A mirror neuron of this type discharges while the animal is observing the experimenter place food on a surface as well as when it picks up the food. There has not been much discussion on the functional role and theoretic significance of these neurons. It is however quite possible that their behaviour is a consequence of the chain organization of motor acts that we will discuss in the last paragraph of this chapter. Taking into consideration the various typologies, the broadly congruent neurons represent approximately 70% of the mirror neurons in the monkey.

Ingestion and communication

So far we have limited our examples to cases involving mirror neurons that are activated by hand movements. Basically, the first studies concentrated almost exclusively on the dorsal region of F5 in which the majority of movements represented are linked to the hand. In the first chapter, we mentioned how electric micro-stimulation and recordings of single neuron activity showed that mouth movements are also controlled in the ventral region of F5. Recent studies have provided evidence that the neurons in this area possess visuo-motor properties that are typical of mirror neurons, responding as they do to the effective execution of motor acts by the mouth and to the observation of similar acts performed by others.[3]

Figure 4.4 illustrates some of the actions performed by the experimenter and the monkey to assess the specificity of the motor and visual responses of the neurons recorded in the animal. The top and centre panels show two typical transitive gestures (i.e. object-related gestures) involving the ingestion of solids or liquids, while the images in the bottom panel show an intransitive act (protrusion of the lips) which, with others such as lip smacking or teeth grinding, belong to the monkey's repertoire of communicative behaviour.

The majority of mirror neurons (approximately 85%) respond to the sight of acts such as grasping a piece of food with the mouth, chewing or sucking it. They have been called *ingestive neurons*. From a functional point of view these neurons are similar to the mirror neurons of the hand: in fact, they too discharge only when the body part interacts with an object; the mere sight of an object or the execution

---

[3] Ferrari *et al.* (2003).

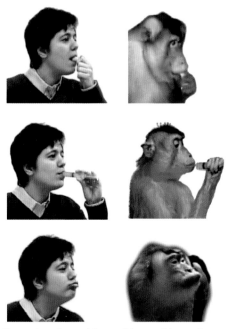

Fig. 4.4 Examples of transitive and intransitive actions performed by experimenter and monkey, used to study the mirror neurons of the mouth. From top to bottom: grasping a piece of food with the mouth, sucking orange juice from a syringe; protrusion of the lips. (Ferrari et al., 2003.)

of an intransitive gesture does not produce any significant response. In addition, most of them are selective to a particular type of act and approximately one-third are strictly congruent (Figure 4.5).

Mirror neurons that respond to the sight of communicative acts carried out with the mouth behave differently. Two examples are given in Figure 4.6; in the first, the experimenter smacks his lips (A), protrudes his lips (B), and sucks from a syringe (C). Only (A) produces a significant response.

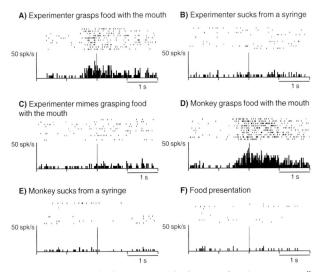

Fig. 4.5 Example of a "grasping-with-the-mouth-mirror-neuron". A. The experimenter moves his mouth close to a piece of food on a stand and grips it with his teeth. B. The experimenter moves his mouth close to a syringe containing juice, resting on a stand, and sucks the juice. C. The experimenter mimes the same action as in A, but without the food. D. The experimenter moves the food close to the monkey, who grasps it with its teeth and eats it. E. The experimenter moves the syringe with the juice close to the monkey, who, after closing its lips around the syringe, sucks the juice. F. The experimenter puts food on a rod and brings the rod into the monkey's field of vision. Each panel shows a series of ten trials and their relative histograms. Test and histograms are aligned to the moment in which the mouths of the experimenter (visual response) and the monkey (motor response) touch the food and to the moment in which the food enters the monkey's visual field. In C. the alignment is with the end of the movement. Ordinates: spikes/s; abscissa: time. Bin size = 20 ms. (Ferrari et al., 2003.)

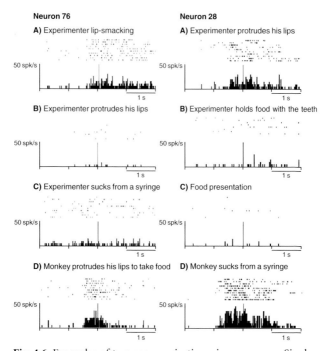

Fig. 4.6 Examples of two communicative mirror neurons. Single trial responses and histograms were aligned with the peak of the action. Neuron 76: (A) The experimenter smacks his lips in front of the monkey. (B) The experimenter protrudes his lips. (C) The experimenter moves his mouth close to a syringe containing juice and sucks the contents. (D) The experimenter offers food to the monkey, who protrudes his lips and grasps it. Neuron 28: (A) The experimenter protrudes his lips while looking at the monkey. (B) The experimenter moves his mouth close to a piece of food placed on a stand, grasps it and holds it between his teeth. (C) The experimenter moves a rod with some food on it in front of the monkey. (D) The experimenter offers the syringe with the juice to the monkey who sucks the juice. (Ferrari et al., 2003.)

However, the same neuron becomes active when the animal grasps food with its mouth, and in doing so, slightly protrudes its tongue and lips (D). In the second example the experimenter protrudes his lips (A), holds food between his teeth (B), and offers it to the monkey (C): in this case too the neuron becomes active only in condition (A), and, as in the previous example, it also discharges when the monkey executes a typically ingestive act, such as sucking juice from a syringe (D).

It should be noted that, unlike the other mirror neurons, *communicative neurons* respond to the sight of intransitive acts. It could be objected that this response does not concern the visual stimulus as such, but rather the monkey's interpretation of it as an ingestive act. In other words, the act of simple tongue protrusion by the experimenter would evoke the motor representation of licking in the monkey. This explanation is appealing only because it unites the mirror neurons in a single theoretical design. Unfortunately, however, it is not compatible with the fact that the observation of ingestive acts produces little, if any, response in the communicative mirror neurons.

An important issue remains to be clarified: unlike the mirror neurons that are linked to hand motor acts and the ingestive neurons, communicative neurons show no congruence between visual and motor responses. Only the former are communicative in nature, while the latter are ingestive. If we take the purely motor aspects, there is generally a good level of correlation between the observed act and the executed act: the neuron that discharges while observing labial protrusion responds to those acts performed by the monkey that require similar movements (sucking juice from the syringe, for example), but not to others, and the same is true for lip smacking. It must be remembered, however, that

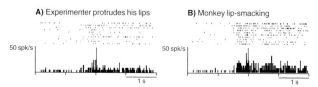

Fig. 4.7 Example of a communicative mirror neuron coding labial protrusion. (A) The experimenter protrudes his lips while looking at the monkey. (B) The monkey responds to the experimenter's lip smacking by smacking its lips. (Ferrari et al., 2003.)

the significance of these acts differs. It is no easy task to persuade a monkey to carry out communicative gestures in an experiment to record single neurons. However in the rare cases in which this has been possible, a clear neuron response linked to the communicative gesture was found (Figure 4.7). This finding would lead us to believe that this would be true for many neurons and not just for a few.

Leaving aside the difficulties encountered in experimental conditions, the fact that the acts of ingestion and communication have a common neural substrate is particularly interesting, especially in the light of certain ethologic studies carried out with non-human primates.[4] Communicative actions such as lip smacking or labial protrusion have evolved from a repertoire of movements which were originally associated with ingestion and linked to grooming. It is well known that among the non-human primates, grooming is one of the principal ways of affiliation and social cohesion: it promotes the formation of groups, and once these become too large, encourages the creation of coalitions within the various groups with the function of protecting the weaker members from aggression by other animals.

---

[4] See Van Hoof (1962;1967); but also Maestripieri (1996).

When a monkey starts to clean and remove fleas from the fur of another monkey, it often accompanies or precedes its first movements with lip smacking. Feeding is also accompanied by lip smacking, but with a lower tone than when grooming, almost as if the monkey wishes to underline the difference between the two acts. Lip smacking without grooming therefore appears to be a *form of ritualized motor act* that transforms object-related functions into communicative functions, and the same holds true for gestures such as labial or tongue protrusion. In this perspective the discovery of communicative mirror neurons in an area such as F5, together with the apparent lack of congruence between the visual and motor responses, would appear to reflect an initial corticalization process of communicative functions that have not yet been completely separated from their ingestive origins (i.e. the transitive action of carrying food to the mouth and ingesting it).

The connections with the superior temporal sulcus and the inferior parietal lobule

As we have seen in Chapter 2, most of the visual information sent to the canonical F5 neurons comes from the anterior intraparietal area (AIP). Now the question is which cortical regions supply the mirror neurons with sensory input.

Over fifteen years ago David I. Perrett and his co-workers[5] demonstrated that in monkeys, the anterior part of the superior temporal sulcus (STS) contained neurons which respond selectively to the sight of a wide range of body movements performed by another individual: some become active when the monkey observes head or eye movements,

---

[5]   See Perrett *et al.* (1989;1990).

others respond to the observation of movements of the trunk and legs (walking), and others again code specific hand–object interactions.

The visual properties of the neurons of this latter group appear to be very similar to those of the F5 mirror neurons. Both neural populations code, to a great extent, the same types of actions observed, with various levels of abstraction (for example, grasping with the hand, grasping with a precision grip, etc.) and do not discharge when observing the experimenter making intransitive movements or mimicking an effective transitive action in the absence of an object. There is however one substantial difference: unlike F5 mirror neurons, STS neurons are purely visual neurons, which do not become active in association with movements. They therefore lack the visuo-motor combination that is the essential characteristic of mirror neurons.

STS neurons are extremely interesting, not only for their properties, but because they allow us to understand how it was possible for neurons as complex as mirror neurons to appear. They show how the encoding of biological movements executed by others takes place in a specific system and how the process of identification of those movements starts in the visual system. It is a simple step then, to assume that the visual information is sent to the motor areas, thus attributing complex visual properties to motor neurons.

The next question is how information is conveyed from STS to F5? From an anatomical point of view, STS does not project directly to the ventral premotor cortex. It is however strongly connected to the inferior parietal lobule and sectors of the prefrontal lobe.[6] The visual information regarding

6 Selzer and Pandya (1994).

observed actions can therefore reach F5 by one of these two paths. It is likely that the latter is less important: it is in fact known that the connections between F5 and the prefrontal lobe that receive information from STS are not very strong; on the other hand, F5 is strongly connected with the rostral part of the inferior parietal lobule which is formed by the areas PF and PFG.[7]

Moreover, the functional properties of the PF–PFG neurons would appear to indicate that the PF–PFG complex may be considered as a bridge between STS and F5. The work by Jari Hyvärinen[8] and his colleagues in the 1980s showed that the neurons belonging to this complex respond to sensory (somatosensory and visual) stimuli and that approximately one-third of them also became active during voluntary movements of the hand and mouth. Later studies[9] show however that approximately 40% of the neurons which respond to visual stimuli become active during the observation of motor acts performed with the hand, such as grasping, holding, reaching, and what is even more important, the majority (approximately 70%) possess motor properties, responding when the monkey carries out actions with its hand, mouth, or both. These are the *parietal mirror neurons*.

Like F5 neurons, parietal mirror neurons do not discharge at the mere sight of an agent or an object, or even when an action is mimed. Half are selective for only one type of motor act and the other half for two (grasping and letting go, for example). With regards the relation between

---

[7] See Petrides and Pandya (1984), among others; Matelli *et al.* (1986). The reader will find further detail relative to this point in the first chapter of this book.

[8] Leinonen *et al.* (1979); Leinonen and Nyman (1979); Hyvärinen (1981). See also Graziano and Gross (1995).

[9] Fogassi *et al.* (1998); Gallese *et al.* (2002).

observed and executed acts, they behave as F5 mirror neurons: some are strictly congruent, but the majority are broadly congruent.

The function of the mirror neurons

Now we must clarify the functional role of the mirror neurons recorded in the F5 and PF–PFG areas. At a superficial glance, we might attribute the activation of these neurons while the monkey is observing actions being carried out by another individual (in our case, the experimenter) to non-specific factors (such as attention or food expectancy), or to a preparation to act that ensures the animal will replicate the gestures it is seeing as rapidly as possible in order to have an edge on any rivals that may be in its vicinity. If this were the case, the mirror neurons would either be devoid of any specific functionality or would simply represent a particular category of those 'preparatory neurons' that are widespread in the premotor cortex and which become active prior to the effective execution of the movement.

A closer look shows that neither of these hypotheses is acceptable. The selectivity of the responses and the visuo-motor congruence found in the majority of mirror neurons cannot be ascribed to animal behaviour related to expectancy of food or other forms of reward. The experiment described in Figure 4.8 provides evidence of this. In (A) and (B) the monkey whose neurons were being recorded, watched another monkey or the experimenter pick up food with their hands; in (C) the monkey itself executes the same action. The mirror neuron discharges in both (A) and (B) in spite of the fact that in both these conditions the monkey could not reach the food and did not receive any reward.

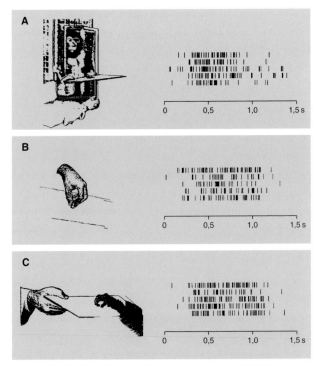

Fig. 4.8 Activation of a 'grasping-mirror-neuron'. (A) The monkey from which the neuron was being recorded watches another monkey, shown in the figure, who picks up food with its hands; (B) The monkey watches the experimenter picking up the food; (C) The monkey executes the same action. Each panel shows 5 trials. The neuron had virtually no spontaneous activity (Rizzolatti et al., 1996a.)

The activity of mirror neurons cannot be satisfactorily explained as a form of preparation to act. In Figure 4.8 it can be seen that when the first monkey observed the other picking up the food, it had no reason to prepare to act, as the food was outside its reach. Moreover, the reader will recall that at no time in the previous experiments did the mirror neurons become active at the sight of a motor act followed by its execution. We must not forget that the mirror neurons never became active when food was offered to the monkey from a distance at which the animal could reach it. Had their response been linked to the preparation of an action, they should have been active during the phase prior to the monkey's execution of the movement.

Some years ago Marc Jeannerod, in an article on motor imagery, proposed a different (and more sophisticated) interpretation of the function of mirror neurons.[10] Imagine a classroom and a pupil who is attentively watching his maestro playing a complicated passage on the violin that he will be required to replicate when the maestro has finished playing. To do this, he must construct a motor image of the rapid movements of the maestro's hands and fingers. Now, according to Jeannerod, the same neurons that are responsible for the production of this motor image will become active during the pupil's preparation and execution of the piece. In other words, the activation of the mirror neurons will generate an 'internal motor representation' of the observed motor act, on which the possibility of learning by imitation relies.

Jeannerod's suggestion is of great value and is in line with the experimental data that we have seen earlier. The close link between the visual and motor responses of the mirror neurons does seem to indicate that when an individual observes an action performed by others, a potential motor act is evoked in his brain which is to all effects similar to that which was spontaneously activated during the organization

---

[10] Jeannerod (1994).

and effective execution of that action. The difference is that while in one case the act remains at the potential stage (as an 'internal motor representation'), in the other it is translated into a concrete sequence of movements. There is one point however on which we cannot agree with Jeannerod: we do not believe that the primary function of the mirror neurons is linked to imitative behaviour.

In the following pages, we will analyse in greater depth the wide range of phenomena which are often considered as–and sometimes confused with–imitation; we will also assess to what extent the capacity of human beings to learn how to perform an action after having seen it executed by others depends on the mirror neuron system. In any case, in recent years ethologists are increasingly of the opinion that imitation in the true sense of the word is the prerogative of humans and (possibly) anthropomorphous apes, but not of the macaques studied in the experiments we have described.[11] Therefore we cannot fully agree with Jeannerod's inter-pretation: the function of the F5 and the PF–PFG complex mirror neurons has an earlier developmental origin and, on the basis of the examples given, it can be said that these neurons are primarily involved in the *understanding of the meaning of 'motor events', i.e. of the actions performed by others*.[12]

Our use of the term 'understanding' does not necessarily mean that the observer (in our case, the monkey) has explicit or even reflexive knowledge that the action seen and the action executed are identical or similar. What we are saying is much simpler: we are referring to the ability to

---

[11]   See Byrne (1995); Tomasello and Call (1997); Visalberghi and Fragaszy (1990;2002) among others.

[12]   di Pellegrino *et al.* (1992).

immediately recognize a specific type of action in the observed 'motor events', a specific type of action that is characterized by a particular modality of interacting with objects; to differentiate that type of action from another, and finally, to use this information to respond in the most appropriate manner. Therefore what was said earlier regarding the F5 canonical neurons and the visuo-motor neurons of the anterior intraparietal area (AIP) holds true in this case also: the visual stimulus is immediately coded starting from the corresponding motor act, even if it is not effectively executed. There is only one, important, difference: in the case of mirror neurons the visual stimulus is not constituted by an object or its movements, but by object-related movements made by another individual with the goal of grasping, holding, or manipulating them. As with objects, these movements take on meaning for the observer, thanks to the vocabulary of motor acts which regulates his own capacity to execute an action. In the case of the monkey, such movements include grasping food, holding it, carrying it to the mouth, and so on: this is why, when it sees the experimenter shaping his hand into a precision grip and moving it towards the food, it immediately *perceives the meaning* of these 'motor events' and *interprets them* in terms of an *intentional act*.

Visual representation and motor understanding of action

There is, however, an obvious objection to this: as discussed above, neurons which respond selectively to the observation of the body movements of others, and in certain cases to hand–object interactions, have been found in the anterior region of the superior temporal sulcus (STS). We have mentioned that the STS areas are connected with the visual, occipital, and temporal cortical areas, so forming a circuit which is in many ways parallel to that of the ventral stream (see Figure 2.7). What point would there be, therefore, in proposing a mirror neuron system that would code in the observer's brain the actions of others in terms of his own motor act? Would it not be much easier to assume that understanding the actions of others rests on purely visual mechanisms of analysis and synthesis of the various elements that constitute the observed action, without any kind of motor involvement on the part of the observer?

Perrett and colleagues[13] demonstrated that the visual codification of actions reaches levels of surprising complexity in the anterior region of the STS. Just as an example, there are neurons which are able to combine information relative to the observation of the direction of the gaze with that of the movements an individual is performing. Such neurons become active only when the monkey sees the experimenter pick up an object on which his gaze is directed. If the experimenter shifts the direction of his gaze, the observation of his action does not trigger any neuron activity worthy of notice. However, we must ask whether this selectivity—or, in more general terms, the capacity to connect different visual aspects of the observed action—is sufficient to justify using the term 'understanding'. The motor activation characteristic of F5 and PF–PFG adds an element that hardly could be derived from the purely visual properties of STS—and without which the association of visual features of the action would at best remain casual, without any unitary meaning for the observer.

---

[13] Jellema *et al.* (2000;2002).

From a motor point of view, the link between the act of reaching for something and the direction of the gaze is certainly not accidental: we learn in the cot that the best way of obtaining an object is to stare at it. Like all successful strategies, this has become part of our vocabulary of acts and so, when we see someone replicating this action our motor system goes into *resonance* mode, by which we recognize the intentional aspect of the movements and understand the type of action.

The visuo-motor properties of the mirror neurons enable them to coordinate *visual information* with *motor knowledge*. The activation of mirror neurons as motor neurons during an action is distinguished not only by the fact that they code type, modality, and timing of the action but that they also control its execution. Now, there cannot be a motor control process without an anticipation mechanism, and therefore every control process determines a correlation between a certain neural activity and the effects this produces. In the specific case of the F5 and PF–PFG areas, the *convalidation* of these effects generates a *basic motor knowledge* of the meanings of the acts coded by the various neurons—knowledge that can be used both during the execution of the action and when observing the action being carried out by others. The activation of the same neural pattern shows that *understanding* the actions of others presumes that the observer possesses the same knowledge of motor principles that regulates the execution of his own actions.

Some recent experiments support the hypothesis that this motor knowledge plays a fundamental role in processing sensory information, to the extent that it would be difficult to talk about *action understanding* without it.[14]

---

[14]   Umiltà *et al.* (2001).

Maria Alessandra Umiltà and colleagues have shown that most F5 neurons respond to actions performed by the experimenter, independently of the fact that in the final phase (i.e. the crucial stage at which hand and object interact) they were hidden from the monkey. Figure 4.9 illustrates their experiment. Single neurons were recorded in four different conditions: in (A) the monkey observes what the experimenter is doing, and has a full view of the final part of the action (the prehension of the object); in (B) it only sees the beginning of the action as the final part is hidden by a screen; in (C) and (D) the conditions are similar to (A) and (B) but the experimenter simply mimes the action, no object is present.

The recordings show that the fact that the monkey was not able to see the final part of the action in no way modified the activation of the neuron with respect to the condition in which the experimenter's hand was fully visible. In condition (B) the monkey had seen the object being placed behind the screen. The neuron's response cannot, however, be interpreted just as a 'reminiscence of the object' because, in that case, the discharge should have begun when the object came into view and this was not the case. On the contrary, the behaviour of the neuron indicates that the same potential motor act occurs when the monkey watches the entire action as when it observes only a part. It is in fact this potential motor act (the 'internal motor representation') that allows the monkey to integrate the missing part of the observed action, recognizing its overall meaning in the partial sequence seen.

A study by Evelyn Kohler and colleagues[15] provided further evidence to support the hypothesis that mirror neuron discharge reflects the meaning of the observed action and

---

[15]   Kohler *et al.* (2002); see also Keynes *et al.* (2003).

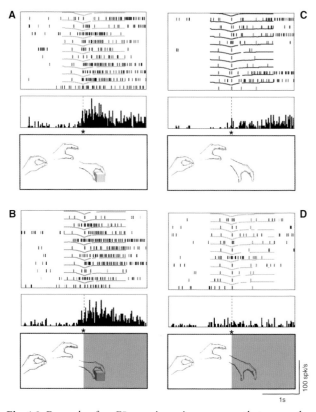

Fig. 4.9 Example of an F5 grasping mirror neuron that responds when hand grasping is not visible. The bottom part of each panel shows the action being performed by the experimenter, as observed from the monkey's viewpoint. In (A) and (B) the experimenter moves his hand towards the object and grasps it. In (C) and (D) he mimes the action. The experiment consists of two basic conditions: view of the grasping hand (A) and (C) and view of arm reaching, but not of grasping (B) and (D). In (B) and (D) the stippled area indicates the screen which blocks the monkey's view of the experimenter' hand. The upper portion of each panel shows the neuron responses and relative histograms recorded during the corresponding movements of the

does not depend simply upon its visual features. The authors individuated a particular type of bimodal F5 mirror neuron (*audio-visual neurons*), which becomes active both when the monkey observes the experimenter carrying out a sound-producing action and when it hears the sound without seeing the action.

Figure 4.10 illustrates the behaviour of two of these neurons: not only are they selective for a particular act (breaking a peanut, for example), but their responses in the diverse experimental conditions (vision and sound, vision only, sound only, and motor execution) are clearly congruent. This means that the potential motor act evoked is always the same, while the sensory information can change depending on the situation. The visual aspects of the action appear to be relevant only to the extent that they facilitate comprehension, but if the action can be understood through other factors (such as sound), the mirror neurons are able to code the experimenter's action even in the absence of visual stimuli.

The melody of action and intention understanding

This demonstration that the mirror neurons of F5 and PF–PFG underlie the understanding of the actions of others should not be interpreted as implying that this is the only

experimenter's hand. The vertical line indicates the point at which the hand of the experimenter activated a photocell that, in the obscured condition, marked the point where the experimenter's hand started to disappear behind the screen. Note the similarity of neuron responses in conditions (A) and (B), and its virtual absence in (C) and (D). (Umiltà et al., 2001.)

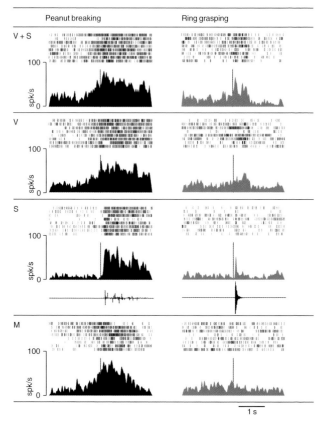

Fig. 4.10 Two 'audio-visual' F5 mirror neurons. The vertical lines in the histograms indicate the onset of sound emission in the vision and sound (V+S) and sound only (S) conditions; in the vision only condition (V), they indicate the point when the sound would have been emitted, if the auditory stimulus had been present, and, finally, in the motor condition they indicate the instant when the monkey touches the object. (Kohler et al., 2003.)

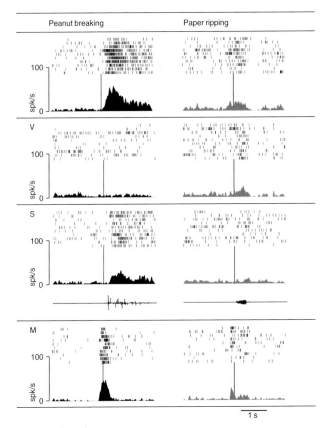

Fig. 4.10 (*cont.*)

function of the mirror mechanism. In the following pages, we will illustrate the range of the mirror neuron functions and provide a map of the cortical areas involved in them for both human and non-human primates. However, this in no way changes the importance of the action understanding mediated by the F5 and PF–PFG neurons and marked by the congruence of their sensory–motor responses. This, as we have seen, is a form of implicit understanding of pragmatic, and not reflexive, origin; it is not constrained by a specific sensory modality, but is bound to the vocabulary of acts which regulates and controls motor execution.

Therefore it is of no consequence if the visual information is partially or even totally substituted with auditory stimuli. Even if it were complete or extremely sophisticated as is the information coded by the STS neurons, it would still be lacking that *motor significance* which can only be obtained through the mutual connection of the PF–PFG and F5 neurons, by which movements performed by others and seen or heard by the observer acquire for him the specific meaning of goal-directed, i.e. intentional motor acts. Thus motor knowledge of our own acts is a necessary and sufficient condition for an immediate understanding of the acts of others. As will be shown in the following paragraphs, this knowledge is of fundamental importance for building a basic intentional cognition because it concerns not only the individual motor acts considered so far, such as grasping, holding, tearing, but also the concatenations of these motor acts into more complex actions.

This aspect of motor organization has recently been studied by Leonardo Fogassi and his colleagues[16], who have recorded a series of parietal mirror neurons (Figure 4.11 A) that became active when the monkey grasped an object. Their experiment had two conditions: in the first, the monkey moved its hand from a pre-established point to grasp a piece of food positioned in front of it, and then carried the food to its mouth; in the second condition, the starting position of the hand was the same, but instead of

[16]   Fogassi *et al.* (2005).

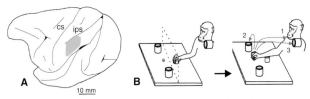

Fig. 4.11 (A) Lateral view of the brain of a monkey showing (shadowed area) the part of the inferior parietal lobe recorded in the study; (B) the experimental paradigm. The container was placed either near the food or on the shoulder. As the speed of the movement required to reach/grasp the food was influenced by the subsequent motor act, by varying the position of the container (and consequently the kinematics of the movement) it was possible to discriminate whether the selectivity of the neurons depends on kinematic factors or the action goal. The results of the experiments demonstrated that it was, in fact, the goal that determined the selectivity of the neurons. (Fogassi et al., 2005.)

carrying the food to its mouth, the monkey placed it in a container (Figure 4.11 B).

The results of these experiments showed that the majority of the neurons recorded in the study discharged differentially depending on whether the motor act following the grasping of the food consisted in carrying the food to the mouth or placing it in a container (see Table 4.1).

Table 4.1 Inferior parietal lobe neurons studied during grasping the food to carry it to the mouth or to place it in the container

Neurons influenced by the goal of the action		
Carry to mouth > Place	Place > Carry to mouth	
77 (72.6%)	29 (27.4%)	106 (64.2%)
Neurons not influenced by the goal of the action		
Carry to mouth = Place		59 (35.8%)
Total		**165 (100%)**

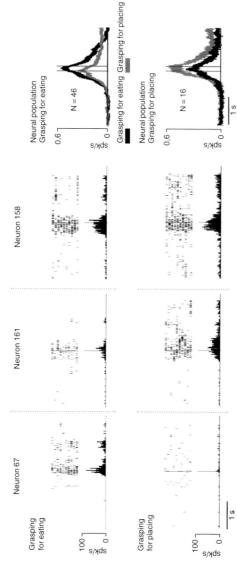

Fig. 4.12 Left: activity of three neurons of the inferior parietal lobe during grasping food to carry it to the mouth and grasping food in order to put it in a container. The individual trials and the histograms are synchronised with the instant when the monkey touched the object to be grasped. The red bars indicate the instant in which the monkey moved its hand from the starting position; the green bars indicate the instant in which the hand touched the food. Right: responses of the neuron population selective for grasping to carry to the mouth (top) and for grasping to place (bottom). The two vertical lines indicate, respectively, the instant in which the monkey touched the container and when grasping was completed. (Fogassi et al., 2005.)

Figure 4.12 illustrates the behaviour of three neurons: it is evident that two discharge differentially according to the type of motor act that follows the act of grasping, while the third codes the grasping independently of the intention that initiated the act.

A series of controls were carried out to verify whether the type of object (food or non-food) or the force with which the object was grasped could explain the selectivity of the neurons for a particular action ('carry to the mouth' or 'move from one point to another'). These alternative interpretations of neuron activity were discarded as a consequence of these controls. In addition, the study of the kinematics (speed, acceleration, etc.) of the reaching/grasping movements showed that the motor parameters characterizing the motor act execution do not influence the selectivity of the various neurons for a particular action.

The reader may feel that it goes against the grain to assume that parietal motor neurons are dedicated to a specific action. Is it not rather excessive to have 'grasping-neurons' exclusively for particular actions? Would it not be more economical to be able to interchange them indiscriminately whenever grasping is required? The answer to these considerations is to be found in a fundamental characteristic of motor organization: fluidity of motion, an aspect that is typical of human actions and those of many animals. The neural organization we have just described appears to have all the necessary requisites to achieve this fluidity. The 'grasping-neurons' are inserted in pre-formed chains that code the entire action, in such a way that each neuron codes the grasping, but is also connected to the successive motor act, guaranteeing fluidity of the action.

However, perhaps an even more interesting aspect of the study carried out by Fogassi *et al.* is that a form of selectivity similar to motor selectivity emerged when the monkey simply observed the experimenter performing the same chain of acts. In this case too, the neurons discharged differentially depending on the type of action in which the motor act they coded was embedded. Moreover these selective neurons also showed a clear congruence between their motor and visual responses (Table 4.2, Figures 4.13 and 4.14).

It is worth noting that in both cases, when the monkey was effectively executing the action and when it was watching actions performed by the experimenter, the neurons became active as soon as the hand (of the monkey or the experimenter) assumed the shape necessary to grip the food or the object. Indeed it is not particularly surprising that the neurons code the intentional meaning of the action during its execution from the very first movement. When the monkey moves its hand in the direction of the food, it already knows if it is going to carry the food to its mouth or move it from one place to another: even if its intention becomes overt only in full deployment of the motor behaviour, it necessarily shapes the initial motor act. In addition, the motion that motor acts are organized into specific motor chains is also supported by the organization of the somatosensory receptive fields of the parietal neurons. The fact that many parietal neurons which

Table 4.2 Inferior parietal lobe neurons studied during the observation of grasping the food to carry it to the mouth or to place it in the container

Neurons influenced by the goal of the action		
Carry to mouth > Place	Place > Carry to mouth	
23 (74.2%)	8 (25.8%)	31 (75.6%)
Neurons not influenced by the goal of the action		
Carry to mouth = Place		10 (24.4%)
Total		**41 (100%)**

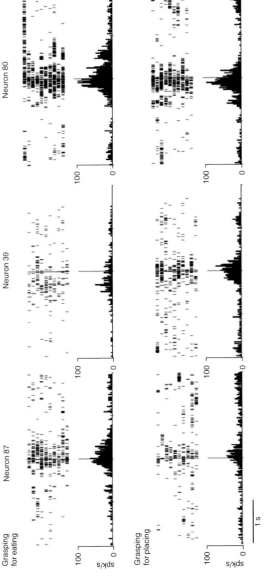

Fig. 4.13 Visual responses of three parietal mirror neurons (Neuron 87, 39 and 80) while the monkey is watching the experimenter grasp food with the aim of eating it or to put it into the container. Neuron 87 discharges with high intensity while the monkey observes the experimenter grasping the food to carry it to his mouth; the response is much weaker when he put it into the container. Neuron 39 behaves in the opposite manner. There is no particular difference in the responses of Neuron 80 in the two conditions. (Fogassi et al., 2005.)

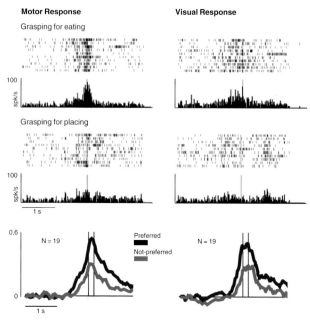

Fig. 4.14 Upper part of the figure. Congruence between the visual and motor responses of a parietal mirror neuron. The discharge of the neuron is stronger during the act of grasping to carry the food to the mouth as opposed to when it grasps it for placing. This occurs both when the monkey carries out the action itself and when it watches the experimenter performing the same action. (Fogassi et al., 2005.). Lower part of the figure. Population-averaged responses during motor and visual tasks.

respond to the passive flexion of the forearm have tactile receptive fields located around the mouth is evidence of this: these neurons would appear to facilitate the opening of the mouth when the animal grasps and lifts an object.[17]

The situation changed when the monkey saw the experimenter's hand grasping the piece of food or another object.

---

[17]   Other examples are to be found in Yokochi et al. (2003).

However, the fact that the visual stimulus activated the same neural pattern—i.e. the same set of potential motor acts that are responsible for the execution of the entire motor chain—shows how the monkey was immediately able to grasp the tangible intentional dynamics of the observed action, anticipating what would be the outcome of the experimenter's action from his very first movements. It is true that there were indications which allowed the monkey to select the appropriate meaning for the motor acts it saw, but if these indications were not available divinatory powers would be needed! The container was one of the most important clues: if it was present, the experimenter put the food in it, if not, he carried it to his mouth. The clues could also interact one with another: in fact, many of the neurons which responded when the monkey observed the act of grasping the food to carry it to the mouth also became active, although weakly, when it observed the act of grasping to place the food (but this was not the case for three-dimensional solids). It was almost as if the presence of food and the sight of a hand approaching it were sufficient to activate, albeit weakly, the chain of acts that would result in the food being carried to the mouth, even though the context indicated that it was more likely that the outcome would be the placing of the food. The responses of other neurons diminished as the action was repeated, as if the activation of the 'grasping-for-placing' chain progressively inhibited that of the 'grasping-for eating' chain.

Taken overall, this confirms the importance of motor knowledge for action understanding, at the same time extending its role and function. Such knowledge allows us to recognize the meaning of the motor acts we observe both when they are performed singly and when they are part of motor chains. In this latter case, their meaning is no longer univocally determined by the specific object relations that differentiate one act from another. Grasping is no longer just grasping, but grasping *for* eating or placing: here the intention to act exceeds the single act and modifies its meaning in the one sense or the other. If the motor chains were not organised as Fogassi and his colleagues have demonstrated, it would be most unlikely that the monkey's brain could release instructions that would result in the fluidity of movement similar, as Alexandr Romanovic Lurija liked to put it, to real 'kinetic melodies'.[18] Moreover, without the mirror properties of those neurons the monkey would not have been able to *catch in a flash*, so to speak, the intention which animated those melodies when they were executed by others, nor would it have been able to anticipate from the very first movements, both the partial result (e.g. grasping the food with the hand), and, more importantly, the complete outcome (e.g. grasping to eat or grasping to place). The clearer the information provided by the context and the object, the more selective was the activation of the pertinent potential motor chains. However, even when the sensory stimuli were ambiguous as they often are (and not only in experimental contexts), the activation of one or more intentionally connected potential motor acts helped the monkey to decipher the experimenter's intentions. The animal was then able to choose the intention that appeared to be most compatible with the scenario, to the point of identifying the most appropriate, and it goes without saying that these deciphering and identification processes were tied to the same motor knowledge that drove and adjusted the animal's execution of the same chain of actions.

---

[18]   Lurija (1973, p. 198).

CHAPTER 5

Mirror neurons in humans

Early evidence

It was a short step from the discovery of mirror neurons in the monkey to the idea that a similar system might exist in the human brain. As often happens (and not only in neurophysiology), discoveries pave the way to a re-reading and re-interpretation of data already present in the literature and this was the case with mirror neurons. Evidence (albeit indirect evidence) supporting the presence of a mechanism which we now interpret as a mirror mechanism was found in EEG (electroencephalography) studies conducted in the early 1950s on the reactivity of cerebral rhythms while observing movement.

It is well known that the EEG records spontaneous cortical electric activities. The EEG rhythms are classified by wave frequency. In healthy adults, at rest and in the eyes-closed condition, the α rhythm (8–12 Hz) dominates the posterior areas of the brain, while the so-called desynchronized rhythms (i.e. high frequency and low voltage) are dominant in the frontal lobe. Another rhythm, known as μ and similar to the α rhythm, is present in the central regions. The α rhythm prevails when the sensory systems, the visual system in particular, are inactive: if the visual condition changes from eyes-closed to eyes-open, this rhythm disappears or weakens considerably. Conversely, the μ rhythm is evident as long as the motor system is at rest; an active movement or a somatosensorial stimulus is needed to desynchronize it.

In 1954 Henri Gastaut[1] and his co-workers conducted experiments that indicated that the μ rhythm is desynchronized not only by the execution of actions but also by the sight of actions carried out by others. Over forty years later, spurred by the discovery of mirror neurons, Vilayanur S. Ramachandran and his co-workers and Stéphanie Cochin and her colleagues[2] repeated these experiments using more refined methodologies. Cochin's group in particular demonstrated that the observation of leg or finger movements was accompanied by a desynchronization of the μ rhythm and that this did not occur when a moving object was shown to the participants. In other words, the same rhythm that was blocked or desynchronized by a movement was also blocked when the movement was observed.

Similar results were obtained from a series of research studies using the MEG (magnetoencephalography), a technique which analyses the electric activity of the brain with recordings of the magnetic fields it generates. These too provided evidence that in the precentral cortex the μ rhythms are desynchronized both during manipulation of an object and when the manipulation is observed.[3]

Transcranial stimulation studies (TMS) provided another very convincing piece of evidence that the human motor system possesses mirror properties. TMS is a non-invasive technique which stimulates the nervous system. A magnetic

---

[1] Gastaut and Bert (1954); Cohen-Seat *et al.* (1954).
[2] Altschuler *et al.* (1997;2000); Cochin *et al.* (1998;1999).
[3] Hari *et al.* (1998).

field emanated by a coil held close to the head induces an electrical current of an appropriate intensity in the motor cortex. This current allows recordings to be taken of the motor potentials (motor evoked potentials or MEPs) in the contralateral muscles. As the size of the MEPs is regulated by the behavioural context, this technique can be used to control the state of excitability of the motor system in various experimental conditions.

Luciano Fadiga and his colleagues[4] recorded the MEPs induced by the stimulation of the left motor cortex in various muscles of the right hands and arms of subjects who were asked to watch an experimenter while he grasped objects with his hand and performed movements that were apparently without meaning and devoid of any connection to an object. In both cases a selective increase in MEPs was found in the recorded muscles while the movements were being observed. Although the increase in MEPs during transitive acts (i.e. object-related acts) was coherent with data collected in studies on monkeys, that noted during intransitive acts (i.e. acts that are not directed towards an object) was somewhat unexpected, considering that the mirror neurons in the monkey do not respond to the sight of non-object-related arm movements.

This is not the only difference between the mirror system in humans and monkeys. Recordings of MEPs in the hand muscles of healthy subjects while watching the experimenter perform typical grasping movements have shown how the activation of the motor cortex faithfully reproduces the temporal duration of the various movements observed; this would seem to suggest that the mirror neurons in

---

[4] Fadiga et al. (1995). See also Maeda et al. (2002).

humans are not only able to code the goal of the motor act, but also the temporal aspects of its individual movements.[5]

Brain imaging studies

The important functional consequences of these findings will be examined later, but before proceeding, there is a further source of evidence for the existence of mirror neurons in humans to be reviewed: brain imaging studies.

While electrophysiological techniques such as EEG, MEG, and the TMS can be used to record specific activations of the human motor system induced by the observation of actions performed by other individuals, they do not precisely localize the cortical areas and the neural circuits involved. Consequently, it is not possible to use them to individuate the overall mirror neuron system architecture. It was therefore necessary to resort to brain imaging methodologies, in particular positron emission tomography (PET) and functional magnetic resonance imaging (fMRI), which allowed the recording of variations in blood flow in the various cerebral regions caused by the performance and observation of specific motor acts.

The first experiment however produced less than satisfactory results.[6] The participants were shown images of grasping movements performed by a hand created in virtual reality. The PET did not record any significant activity in the motor areas that could correspond to the ventral premotor cortex in the monkey; the effects that emerged from the electrophysiological studies mentioned earlier did not seem to have an explanation.

---

[5] Gangitano *et al.* (2001).
[6] Decety *et al.* (1994).

This experiment was later repeated by other researchers[7], but with an important variation: the movements were executed by a real hand and not by a clearly unrealistic virtual image. This time the PET data confirmed the results found in the monkey: there were frontal areas which became active when individuals observed hand actions performed by others. Later fMRI studies provided a more precise localization of the areas involved in the mirror neuron system: the areas constantly activated during action observations are the rostral (anterior) portion of the inferior parietal lobule and the lower part of the precentral gyrus plus the posterior part of the inferior frontal gyrus. In certain experimental conditions a more anterior region of the inferior frontal gyrus and the dorsal premotor cortex were also activated (Figure 5.1).

While it is always risky to interpret information on cortical activity obtained by brain imaging in terms of cytoarchitectonic areas, it is very likely that the region which is activated in the inferior parietal lobule corresponds to Brodmann's area 40, which is the human homologue of the PF area, that, as we saw earlier, is one of the areas where mirror neurons have been found in monkeys. In contrast, the activation of the lower part of the precentral gyrus and of the posterior part of the inferior frontal gyrus is more difficult to localize cytoarchitectonically. For many years it was thought that these were two radically different areas with no functional relationship: the posterior part of the inferior frontal gyrus was held to correspond to Brodmann's area 44 (in other words, to the posterior part of Broca's area), and was thought to be responsible for speech production,

---

[7] Rizzolatti et al. (1996b). See also Grafton et al. (1996); Grèzes et al. (1998;2001).

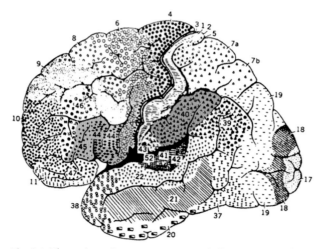

Fig. 5.1 The action mirror neuron system in humans. Lateral view of a human brain showing the cytoarchitectonic areas according to Brodmann. Reddish shaded areas: sector of the parietal lobe that becomes active during action execution and during the observation of actions being performed by others. Yellow shaded areas: sector of the frontal lobe that activates in the same experimental conditions. These two sectors together form the action mirror neuron system. Some authors also include the dorsal area 6 in this system. However activation of this area during observation could be due to preparation to act rather than to true mirror activation. Blue shaded areas: sector of the frontal lobe, which becomes active in certain experimental conditions while watching actions by others. One should be cautious before including this area in the mirror neuron system as, like the region of the superior temporal sulcus, its neurons may lack motor properties. The mirror neuron system illustrated here codifies actions without emotional content. The reader is referred to Chapter 7 for a discussion on actions with emotional content.

while the lower part of the precentral gyrus was classified as part of the motor cortex.

To give credit where credit is due, in the early years of the twentieth century Alfred Walter Campbell, one of the fathers of cytoarchitecture, drew attention to the anatomical analogies between the posterior part of the inferior frontal gyrus and the lower part of the precentral gyrus, coining the term 'intermediate precentral cortex'.[8] His indications, however, were ignored for many years. Only recently have comparative anatomy studies shown that Brodmann's area 44 (or at least a part of it) can be considered as the human homologue of area F5 in the monkey[9]; moreover, it has become increasingly clear that area 44 possesses a representation of the hand and mouth.[10]

Now, can this area be attributed with a key role in the human mirror neuron system on the strength of these findings? Can we really push the functional homology with area F5 in the monkey to the point of interpreting the activation shown in brain imaging studies as evidence that the neurons of the posterior part of the inferior frontal gyrus possess analogous mirror properties? Would it not be easier to hypothesize that their activation reflects an 'internal verbal representation'?[11] We often make mental descriptions of actions we are observing; for example, we may mutter to ourselves 'Just look at that, so and so is taking my cup of coffee!'. Now, can we really exclude that something like this happened to the participants in the PET experiment? After all, it did involve a portion of Broca's area!

[8] Campbell (1905).
[9] Petrides and Pandya (1997).
[10] Krams *et al.* (1998); Binkofski *et al.* (1999); Ehrsson *et al.* (2000).
[11] See Grézes and Decety (2001); Heyes (2001).

Giovanni Buccino and his colleagues[12] took up the challenge to respond to this objection with an fMRI experiment. They asked some students to look at a video in which actors were either executing transitive actions such as biting an apple, picking up a cup of coffee, kicking a football, or miming them. Observation of the transitive mouth movements activated two foci in the frontal lobe—one corresponding to the posterior part of the inferior frontal gyrus and the other in the inferior precentral gyrus—and two in the inferior parietal lobule, while observation of transitive hand movements resulted in a similar activation pattern, although that of the lower part of the precentral gyrus was located in a more dorsal position and that of the rostral part of the inferior parietal lobule was more posterior. Transitive foot movements showed a frontal activation, located in a more dorsal position compared to those recorded during observation of hand and mouth movements, and a further posterior shift of the parietal activation. In other words, although significant overlapping was present, the mirror neuron system was seen to be somatotopically organized, with cortical foci dedicated to hand, mouth, and foot movements. Observation of the mimed actions showed an analogous activation pattern that was however limited to the frontal lobe (Figure 5.2).

If the verbal mediation theory were correct, Broca's area should have activated independently of the type of action observed and the effector used, nor would any activation of the premotor cortex be expected. However, the above results do not support this theory and so, unless we want to

---

[12]   Buccino *et al.* (2001).

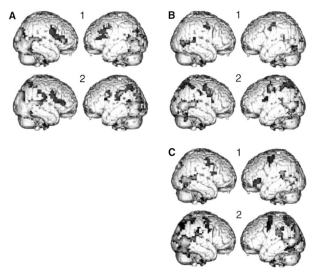

Fig. 5.2 Cortical areas activated during observation of mimed actions (1) and object directed (transitive) actions (2) performed with the mouth (A), hand (B) and foot (C). (Buccino et al., 2001.)

resort to a rather bizarre *ad hoc* explanation, maintaining for example that verbal representation would be present during observation of mouth and hand movements, but would (magically) disappear when foot movements were being observed, we must accept that the activation of Broca's area reflects the typical behaviour of mirror neurons. Moreover, the experiment by Buccino *et al.* shows that the mirror neuron system in humans includes large portions of the premotor cortex and the inferior parietal lobule as well as Broca's area. It also provides evidence that the mirror neuron system is not confined to hand movements and transitive acts alone, but also responds to mime.

Capturing the intentions of others with our mirror systems

We have seen that both electrophysiology and brain imaging studies show that a mirror system analogous to that found in monkeys is also present in humans. There are however some significant differences: the mirror system appears to include more cortical space in humans than in monkeys although this conclusion must be treated with a certain degree of caution given the different experimental techniques used in the different species: it is one thing to record the activity of single neurons, quite another to analyse the activation of the various cortical areas on the basis of variations in blood flow. What is most important, however, is that the human mirror neuron system has certain properties which have not been found in monkeys: for example, it codes both transitive and intransitive motor acts, it is able to code both the goal of the motor act and the movements of which the act is composed, and finally, in the case of transitive actions, effective object interaction is not a mandatory condition as it can activate when the action is merely mimed.

We have already mentioned that these properties can have important functional implications; however, the fact that the human mirror neuron system can accomplish a wider range of tasks than that observed in the monkey must not obscure its *primary* role, i.e. the role linked to *understanding the meaning of the actions of others*. In fact, the TMS experiments have shown that the sight of hand acts performed by others results in an increase in the MEPs recorded in the same hand muscles used by the observer to execute the same acts. On the other hand, brain imaging studies have shown that the activation of the frontal lobe resulting from the observation of acts performed with the hands, mouth, and feet determines activations that basically correspond to the somatotopic motor representation of these body parts.

In humans, as in monkeys, the sight of acts performed by others produces an immediate activation of the motor areas deputed to the organization and execution of those acts, and through this activation it is possible to decipher the meaning of the 'motor events' observed, i.e. to *understand* them in *terms of goal-centred movements*. This understanding is completely devoid of any reflexive, conceptual, and/or linguistic mediation as it is based exclusively on the *vocabulary of acts* and the *motor knowledge* on which our capacity to act depends. Finally, again as in the monkey, this understanding is not limited to single motor acts but extends to entire chains of acts.

This last point emerges very clearly from an fMRI experiment conducted by Marco Iacoboni and colleagues[13], in which three different videos were shown to a number of volunteers (Figure 5.3). In the first video the participants saw a number of objects (a teapot, a mug, a glass, a plate, etc.) laid out on a table as if someone were about to have tea (a change from our usual cup of coffee!) or had just finished. The condition related to this video was called *context* for brevity. The second video showed a hand grasping the mug in a whole-hand prehension or a precision grip without the context (the *action* condition), and the third video showed the same hand with the same prehension forms but this time in context, so as to suggest the intention of picking the mug up to carry it to the lips or to clear it off the table (the *intention* condition).

---

[13] Iacoboni *et al.* (2005).

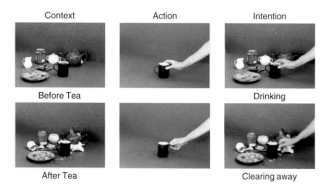

Context	Action	Intention
Before Tea		Drinking
After Tea		Clearing away

Fig. 5.3 Stimuli used to study the cortical areas involved in the comprehension of the intentions of others. The columns show the stimuli used in the three experimental conditions: *context, action, intention*. In the condition *context* (first column) the volunteers saw a table laid for breakfast (above), and the same table after breakfast (below). In the condition *action* (second column) they saw a hand grasping the mug using a whole-hand prehension (above) or a precision grip (below). No context was provided. In the third condition (*intention*), the two types of prehension were shown in the "before" and "after" breakfast contexts suggesting the intention, respectively, of "grasping-the-mug-to-drink" (above) and "grasping-the-mug-to-clear-it-away" (below). (Iacoboni et al., 2005.)

If we compare the cerebral activations induced by observation of the three conditions compared to the *rest* condition (Figure 5.4), we will see that in the *action* and *intention* conditions, activity increased in the visual areas and in the parieto-frontal circuits linked to the encoding of motor acts, while in the *context* condition there was no increase in activity in the regions of the STS (superior temporal sulcus), which responds to moving visual stimuli, nor in the lower parietal lobe, although it was significant in the premotor areas. This may be ascribed to the presence of 'graspable'

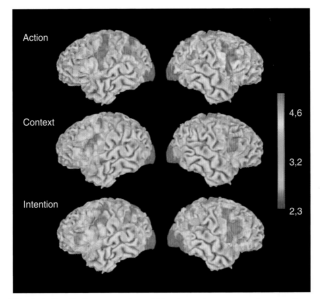

Fig. 5.4 Cortical areas active while observing a scene (context), actions without context (action), actions inserted into context (intention). The colours indicate the active areas, with red indicating where the activity is strongest. (Iacoboni et al., 2005.)

objects activating the canonical neurons, which, as we have seen, respond to *object affordances.*

The most relevant comparisons were those between the *intention* and *action* conditions, and the *intention* and *context* conditions. As can be seen in Figure 5.5, the activation of the dorsal portion of the posterior section of the right inferior frontal gyrus (top section of Figure 5.5) was greater in the *intention* condition than in the other two conditions (*action* and *context*). This is particularly interesting because the activation is localized in the frontal node of the mirror neuron system, which indicates that not only does the mirror neuron system code the observed act (in this

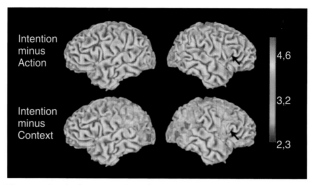

Fig. 5.5 Cortical areas active when viewers try to understand the intentions of others. The upper panel contrasts the areas activated in the *intention* condition (in which the participants try to comprehend, on the basis of a visual context, why an action is being carried out) and the *action* condition (in which they see it being executed but do not have any elements to assist in comprehending why) (*intention minus action*); the lower panel contrasts the areas activated in the intention condition and during the observation of visual scene (*intention minus context*). In both cases the posterior portion of the inferior frontal gyrus is activated. This area, which is part of the mirror neuron system, appears to be greatly involved in the understanding of the intentions of others. (Iacoboni et al., 2005.)

case, grasping a mug with a particular type of grip), it also codes the intention with which the act is performed. This may be because while the observer is watching someone performing a motor act, he is already anticipating possible successive acts in the chain (for example, 'grasp-to-drink' or 'grasp-to-place').

It is interesting to note that observing the act of bringing to the mouth determines greater activity in the mirror neuron system than does the act of grasping to clear away (Figure 5.6).

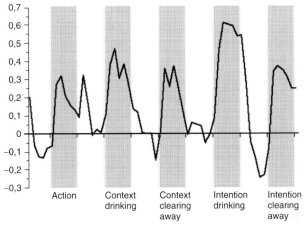

Fig. 5.6 Time series of the right inferior frontal area showing increased signal in the contrast Intention minus Action and Intention minus Context. As shown in the previous figure, this is the area that becomes active when the viewer "reads" the intentions of others. It is interesting to note that observing the act of 'grasping-the mug-to drink" determines more activity in the mirror neuron system than does "grasping-the-mug-to-clear-it-away". (Iacoboni et al., 2005.)

This is in line with the data obtained by Fogassi *et al.* and reported in the previous chapter. Their experiment showed that there were many more neurons coding 'grasping-for-eating' than 'grasping-for-placing'. In addition, even when the sensory information regarding the context (presence of a container) suggested that the act most likely to occur after the 'grasping' was 'placing-the-object-in-the-container', the sight of the experimenter's hand grasping the food activated, however weakly, the chain of neurons responsible for 'grasping-to-carry-the-object-to-the-mouth', as this is the natural sequence in the monkey motor repertoire. In Iacoboni's research, similar results were found; the activation of the inferior right frontal cortex was stronger when the act was 'carrying-the-mug-to-the-mouth-to-drink' than when it entailed 'grasping-the-mug-to-clear-it-away'. It is always the most natural motor intention, most strongly rooted in the basic repertoire of our vocabulary of acts, which tends to prevail.

It goes without saying that, as is the case in motor acts, the activation of mirror neurons is not the only means we have to understand the intentions inherent in the actions of others. Every day we ascribe to others, more or less explicitly, beliefs, desires, expectations, intentions, etc.; our social behaviour depends mostly on our capacity to comprehend what others have in mind and on the conduct we decide to adopt in consequence. At present there is no neural mechanism that explains these mind-reading processes; it might be that they are evolutionarily linked to the mirror neuron system. What counts here, however, is that the mirror neuron mechanism captures the intentional dimension of actions, common to both the agent and the observer. A quotation from Merleau-Ponty is very appropriate here:

> The sense of gesture is not given, but understood, that is, recaptured by an act on the spectator's part. The whole difficult is to conceive this act clearly without confusing with a cognitive operation. The communication or comprehension of gestures comes about through the reciprocity of my intentions and the gestures of others, of my gestures and the intentions discernible in the conduct of other people. It is as if the other person's intentions inhabited my body and mine his. The gestures which I witness outlines an intentional object. This object is genuinely present and fully comprehended when the powers of my body adjust themselves to it and overlap it.[14]

---

[14]   Merleau-Ponty (1945, p. 215).

The 'act on the spectator's part' is a potential motor act, determined by the activation of the mirror neurons that code sensory information in motor terms thus enabling the 'reciprocity' of acts and intentions that is at the root of our ability to immediately understand what we see others doing. The understanding of the intentions of others is not, in this case, based on mentalizing, i.e. on a meta-representative activity, but depends on the selection of those action chains that are most compatible with the observed situation. As soon as we see someone doing something, either a single act or a chain of acts, his movements take on immediate meaning for us, whether he likes it or not. Obviously, the converse is also true: our actions have an immediate value for those who observe them. The mirror neuron system and the selectivity of the responses of the neurons that compose it, produce a *shared space of action*, within which each act and chain of acts, whether ours or 'theirs', are immediately registered and understood without the need of any explicit or deliberate 'cognitive operation'.

Differences in vocabulary

What happens when the movements we observe are not part of our vocabulary of motor acts? In the experiments examined in the preceding chapter, we saw that in the monkey, mirror neurons discharge not only when another monkey is grasping the food but also when it is the experimenter who is performing the act. This is not surprising, given that grasping is present in the monkey's motor vocabulary (as are holding, tearing, pushing, throwing, etc.) All the same, we often see actions that are not part of our motor knowledge; maybe they are not part of the heritage of our species, or, more simply, we just are not able to do them.

Recently, a group of volunteers participating in an fMRI experiment[15] were shown a video, without sound, in which individuals of different species (man, monkey, and dog) performed ingestive (biting) or communicative (talking, lip smacking, barking) acts. Figures 5.7 and 5.8 show stills from these videos.

Although a man biting a piece of food is very different, visually speaking, from a monkey or a dog (even more so), there was a clear overlapping of the cortical areas that became active in the three cases. In fact, watching the three videos produced the activation of two sites (a rostral and a caudal) in the inferior parietal lobule as well as the posterior part of the inferior frontal gyrus and the adjacent precentral gyrus. There was a certain activation asymmetry between the left and right hemispheres in the three cases: in the left hemisphere the response was virtually independent of whether the action was executed by the man, the monkey, or the dog, while in the right hemisphere, on the other hand, the activation was stronger when the action was performed by the man (Figure 5.9).

Activation was completely different when the communicative acts were observed. The sight of a man moving his lips as if he were talking induced strong activation in the posterior part of the inferior frontal gyrus (the region that corresponds to Broca's area); the activation became weaker when the participants watched the monkey lip smacking, and disappeared completely when they watched the dog barking (Figure 5.10).

In purely visual terms, the difference between the various communicative acts would not appear to be greater than

---

[15]   Buccino *et al.* (2004).

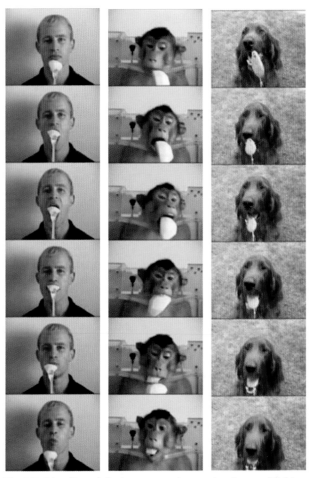

Fig. 5.7 Stimuli used during an experiment aimed at establishing brain activations during the observation of actions that are common to humans and animals. The stills, selected from the video recordings of the experiment, show a man, a monkey and a dog biting a piece of food. (Buccino et al., 2004a.)

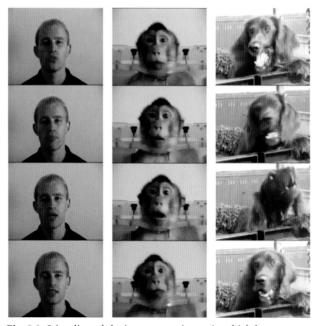

Fig. 5.8 Stimuli used during an experiment in which human communicative gestures were compared with those of other species. The stills, selected from the video recordings of the experiment, show a man, a monkey and a dog in the process of talking, lip smacking and barking, respectively. (Buccino et al., 2004a.)

that which distinguishes the ingestive act of biting as performed by these individuals of the three species, and would therefore not appear to justify the differences found in the activation of the respective neural patterns. The lack of response from the areas of the mirror neuron system during observation of the dog barking cannot simply be ascribed to the type of visual information received. In the previous chapter we have seen that the activity of the mirror

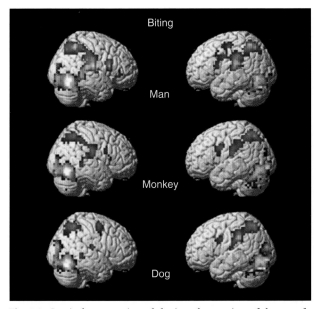

Fig. 5.9 Cortical areas activated during observation of the act of biting a piece of food (see Fig. 5.7) by a man, a monkey and a dog respectively. (Buccino et al., 2004a.)

neurons is not linked to a specific sensory input; it is bound to the vocabulary of acts that regulates the organization and execution of movements. Barking just does not belong to the human vocabulary of motor acts.

Does this mean that we are not able to understand the movements of a dog barking and distinguish them from those it makes when it bites food? Of course not! It simply depends on two different comprehension modalities; the first is based predominantly on visual information, while the other is visuo-motor in nature. When we observe a dog barking, our understanding of this act appears to be linked principally to the activation of the areas localized in the

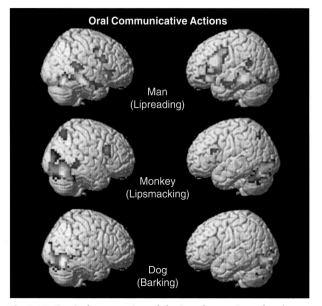

Fig. 5.10 Cortical areas activated during observation of oral communication (see Fig. 5.8) by a man, a monkey and a dog respectively. (Buccino et al., 2004a.)

superior temporal sulcus (STS). These, and other visual areas, also become active when the other (monkey and human) communicative acts are being observed—but in these latter cases the information sourcing from STS activates the potential motor acts coded in the mirror neuron system, by which the meaning of the acts that are being observed are understood immediately.[16]

Similar differences have been found between individuals belonging to the same species. Beatriz Calvo Merino and co-workers[17] conducted an fMRI study which demonstrated

---

[16]   For a comprehensive view of these studies, see Allison *et al.* (2000).
[17]   Calvo-Merino *et al.* (2005).

that cerebral activity may change depending on the specific motor competencies of those who are observing specific actions being performed by others. Their participants, who included classical dancers, teachers of Capoeira, and people who had never taken a dancing lesson in their life, were shown a video of Capoeira and another of classical dance steps. The teachers' mirror neuron system responded most strongly to the sight of the Capoeira steps, while the classical dancers' mirror neuron system responded most strongly to the sight of classical dance steps, compared to those of the Capoeira teachers and, of course, of the beginners.

In a further experiment, these authors tried to understand whether the differences in activation were due to the fact that the teachers of Capoeira had a greater *visual* experience of Capoeira steps in addition to their knowledge of how they should be executed than either the classical dancers or (obviously) the beginners. In Capoeira, some steps can be executed by both men and women, while others are different for the two sexes—obviously all the dancers, men and women, must know the steps that their partner will execute. With this in mind, Calvo Merino and her colleagues showed the Capoeira teachers a video showing steps executed by men and women. They found that the mirror neuron system was activated more strongly by the sight of steps executed by members of the observer's sex, indicating that, in this case, activation was regulated by motor practice and not by visual experience.

Taken together, these experiments confirm the decisive role played by motor knowledge in understanding the meaning of the actions of others. This is not to say that these actions cannot be understood with other means, by intellectual processes based on a more or less sophisticated processing of sensory information in general and visual information in particular, but it does mean that there is a vast difference between these two modalities. Only in the former case does the observed action entail a first person involvement 'on the spectator's part', almost as if he were performing it, thus allowing him to catch its meaning immediately.

The extension and the reach of this 'as if' depends on the motor repertoire of the observer, whether his own, or that of his species. Leo Sperber (son of the better known Dan) put it beautifully when he said: 'Do you know why I don't want to be a dog, Dad? I wouldn't know how to wag my tail!' [18]

---

[18]   Dan Sperber, personal communication.

CHAPTER 6

Imitation and language

Imitation mechanisms

As soon as mirror neurons were discovered, the question raised was whether they might be the neural basis of the ability to imitate. Before examining this possibility, however, we must define exactly what we mean by *imitation*. Anyone who has dabbled in this area knows that over time the term has acquired different and sometimes contrasting meanings in various branches of research (developmental psychology, comparative psychology, ethology, etc.). For the purposes of this book we will narrow the field of possible definitions to two, even at the risk of oversimplification. The first, which is used mainly by experimental psychologists, characterizes imitation as the capacity of an individual to *replicate* an act which already belongs to his motor repertoire, after having seen it executed by others[1]; the second, accepted principally by ethologists, considers imitation to be a process by which an individual *learns* a new pattern of action by observation, after which he is able to reproduce it in minimal detail.[2]

---

[1] See, for example, Bekkering and Wohlschlaeger (2002); Wohlschlaeger *et al.* (2003).

[2] See, for example, Byrne (1995); Tomasello and Call (1997); Visalberghi and Fragaszy (2002).

Albeit in different ways, both notions pose a number of questions that every theory of imitation must face, whatever definition is being assumed. First of all, there are those connected to the so-called *correspondence problem*: how can we actually *do* something we have *seen* others doing? In other words, how can we execute an action similar to that which we have seen others performing, on the basis of observation alone? The coding parameters used by the visual system are different to those used by the motor system. Which therefore are the cortical processes involved and which sensory–motor transformations are required? When we look at the learning process we find that there are further complications: in addition to the correspondence problem, there is also the issue of the *transmission* of competences and motor abilities that in their complexity may not be present in our vocabulary of acts. How do we acquire new actions? How do we translate the sight of a sequence of movements, which taken individually could be devoid of meaning, into a potential action that has sense for us?

We will start with the definition of imitation as the capacity of an individual to replicate an observed act. There are two main theoretical models that have been proposed to explain this ability. The first is based on a clear separation between sensory and motor codes; imitation would be possible due to the associative processes that link elements which, *a priori*, have nothing in common.[3] The second, on the other hand, assumes that the action as observed and as executed must share the same neural code and that this is the *sine qua non* condition for imitation.

---

[3] See, for example, Welford (1968); Massaro (1990).

In recent years, this latter model appears to prevail, thanks principally to the work done by Wolfgang Prinz and his collaborators, which is based on the concept of 'ideomotor action', expounded first by Hermann Lotze and then by William James[4], and extended to imitation under the form of the principle of 'ideomotor compatibility' by the American psychologist Anthony G. Greenwald.[5] On the basis of this principle, the more an act resembles one which is present in the observer's motor repertoire, the greater is the tendency to execute it: perception and execution of

---

[4] Lotze (1852); James (1890). In Chapter XXVI of *his Principles of Psychology*, in which he frequently cites Lotze's *Medicinische Psychologie*, James draws attention to the fact that the majority of our daily actions do not require an *'express resolve'*, an explicit fiat, following *'unhesitatingly and immediately'* the appearance of an idea or a representation-providing that there is no *'conflicting notion in the mind'*: 'We know what it is to get out of bed on a freezing morning in a room without a fire, and how the very vital principle within us protests against the ordeal. Probably most persons have lain on certain mornings for an hour at a time unable to brace themselves to the resolve. We think how late we shall be, how the duties of the day will suffer; we say, "I *must* get up, this is ignominious," etc.; but still the warm couch feels too delicious, the cold outside too cruel, and resolution faints away and postpones itself again and again just as it seemed on the verge of bursting the resistance and passing over into the decisive act. Now how do we *ever* get up under such circumstances? If I may generalize from my own experience, we more often than not get up without any struggle or decision at all. We suddenly find that we *have* got up. A fortunate lapse of consciousness occurs; we forget both the warmth and the cold; we fall into some revery connected with the day's life, in the course of which the idea flashes across us, "Hollo! I must lie here no longer—an idea which at that lucky instant awakens no contradictory or paralyzing suggestions, and consequently produces immediately its appropriate motor effects It was our acute consciousness of both the warmth and the cold during the period of struggle, which paralyzed our activity then and kept our idea of rising in the condition of *wish* and not of *will*. The moment these inhibitory ideas ceased, the original idea exerted its effects.' (James, 1890, p. 793).

[5] Greenwald (1970).

actions must therefore possess a 'common representational domain', this domain being modulated by the observer's understanding of the goal of the movements executed by the demonstrator.[6]

The discovery of mirror neurons suggests a possible reformulation of the *ideomotor compatibility principle*: the *common representational domain* would not be considered as an abstract, amodal domain but rather as a mechanism to transform visual information directly into potential motor acts. This appears to be confirmed by brain imaging studies, of which those conducted by Marco Iacoboni and his colleagues[7] are particularly relevant.

The basic experimental procedures used in those experiments were the following: a fixation point and video clips showing a human hand raising the index or middle finger (A), the same hand, motionless, with a cross marked on either the index or the middle finger (B), and a grey background on which a cross was drawn (C), were shown on a computer screen. The participants were asked simply to observe the stimuli, or, having observed them, to raise the finger they had seen moving on the screen ('imitation') or to raise the finger on which they had seen a cross marked. In a further condition they were told to move their index finger when the cross appeared to the left of the fixation point and their middle finger when the cross appeared to the right. The results showed that during imitation, activation was present in the posterior part of the left inferior frontal gyrus (the so-called frontal pole of the mirror system) as well as the region of the right superior temporal sulcus (STS) and that this activation was stronger than during non-imitative

---

[6] Bekkering *et al.* (2000); Bekkering (2002).
[7] Iacoboni *et al.* (1999; 2001).

motor acts. This difference shows that the mirror system is involved in the imitation of acts already present in the observer's motor repertoire, suggesting an immediate motor translation of the observed action.

Similar results were obtained by Nobuyaki Nishitani and Riitta Hari in MEG experiment[8] in which the participants were asked to grasp an object (A), observe this action being done by the experimenter (B), and observe and replicate the action seen (C). As is well known, MEG is less effective than fMRI from the point of view of spatial resolution; notwithstanding this drawback, however, its excellent temporal resolution picks up the dynamics of the processes under examination. Thus it was seen that in motor condition (A) the left lower frontal cortex (area 44—the frontal node of the mirror system) became active before the hand touched the object, and activation of the left precentral motor area followed after 100–200 ms. During observation (B) and imitation (C), the sequence was similar, but started from the left occipital cortex. Activation was always strongest during action imitation. These results clearly indicate that the left area 44 is strongly involved in action imitation.

It is important to keep in mind that brain imaging data are correlation data; they tell us that certain areas of our brain become active during certain tasks, but what they do not tell us is how important the activated area is for the function being studied. Repetitive transcranial magnetic stimulation (rTMS) does provide this information as it is possible to determine an area's transitory hypofunctionality by lengthy stimulation. This technique has been used recently to verify whether mirror neurons play a crucial role in imitation.[9]

---

[8] Nishitani and Hari (2000); see also Nishitani and Hari (2002).
[9] Heiser *et al.* (2003).

A group of volunteers accepted to have the posterior part of their left frontal gyrus (Broca's area) stimulated while they pressed keys on a keyboard, either while imitating a similar movement executed by another individual or in response to a point of red light which, directed onto the keyboard, indicated which key to press. The data showed that rTMS impaired the participants' performance during imitation, but not during the visuo-motor task. It is interesting to note that the imitative and the non-imitative tasks were identical from a motor point of view.

The above evidence suggests that the mirror neuron system does play a fundamental role in imitation, coding observed actions in motor terms and thus enabling us to replicate them. It is worthwhile here noting that in the experiment conducted by Iacoboni and colleagues, STS area activation was slightly stronger during imitation than during observation. Subsequently, these authors ran a study in which the participants had either to *observe* the movements carried out by the experimenter with his right or left hand or to *replicate* them after observation, but using their *right hand* only; the results obtained showed that not only did activation in the STS area vary according to whether the participant merely observed or also had to imitate, but also depended on the hand used. When observation alone was required, the strongest activation was caused by the movements of the experimenter's hand that corresponded *anatomically* to the hand used by the participants (i.e. the right hand); conversely, during imitation, the strongest activation was caused by the movements of the experimenter's hand that corresponded *spatially* to the hand used by the participants (i.e. the left hand). In other words, when the task was limited to observation, an anatomical congruence prevailed (right hand–right hand) but when the participants were required to imitate the action, the congruence became spatial (*my* right hand, *your* left hand).[10] It is probable that this inversion in the activation of STS during imitation is to be ascribed to the influence of the fronto-parietal mirror neurons, which would promote the selection of motor prototypes that are spatially congruent with those that are being observed. Try telling a friend that he (or she) has a mark on their face and indicate a point on your own right cheek with your right hand: you will see that they will rub their left cheek with their left hand!

Imitation and learning

In the preceding section we have discussed imitation in the first sense of the term; now we must investigate what happens when it is not just the repetition of an act belonging to the observer's motor repertoire but requires the learning of a *new action pattern*. Do mirror neurons play a role in this too?

A number of models have been developed in recent years to explain the mechanisms underlying this form of imitation; of these, particular mention must be made of that presented by Richard Byrne, an ethologist working with the University of St. Andrews. According to Byrne's model, learning by imitation results from the integration of two distinct processes: in the first the observer segments the action to be imitated into its individual elements or, in other words, he converts the continuous flow of movements observed into a string of acts belonging to his motor repertoire; in the second he arranges these coded motor acts into a sequence that will compose an action replicating that of

---

[10]   Iacoboni *et al.* (2001); for similar experiments, see Koski *et al.* (2002; 2003).

the demonstrator.[11] A similar process could also be at the base of learning non-sequential motor patterns, such as notes played on a piano or strummed on a guitar.

This form of learning by imitation was studied by the Parma team in collaboration with experimenters from the Jülich Research Centre. A group of people who had never played a guitar were shown a video clip of the hand of a teacher executing some chords; after a brief interval, they were asked to repeat the chords they had seen.[12] The experimental paradigm also consisted of three control conditions: in the first, the participants touched the neck of the guitar after watching the video, but received specific instructions not to execute any chords; in the second, they were required to fixate the neck of the guitar which was moving to and fro, and then, after a pause, the chord being played by the teacher; in the third condition they were allowed to play a chord of their choice (Figure 6.1).

The mirror neuron circuit was activated when the participants observed the chords with the aim of imitating the teacher; it also became active, though to a lesser extent, during the control conditions when the participants watched the teacher playing the chords or when, after watching the teacher, they touched the neck of the guitar without actually playing the chords themselves (Figure 6.2). The most interesting finding, however, was the intense and extensive activation of the region of the frontal cortex corresponding to Brodmann's area 46 during the pause preceding imitation (Figure 6.3). During the execution of the movement, the motor areas activated independently of whether the task was imitative or not.

---

[11]   Byrne and Russon (1998); Byrne (2002; 2003).
[12]   Buccino *et al.* (2004b).

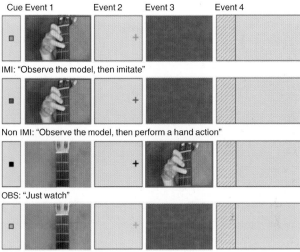

Cue Event 1   Event 2   Event 3   Event 4

IMI: "Observe the model, then imitate"

Non IMI: "Observe the model, then perform a hand action"

OBS: "Just watch"

ExE: "Play a chord of your choice"

Fig. 6.1 Signal. Event 1, Event 2, Event 3, Event 4. IMI: "observes the model and imitates"; Not IMI: "observes the model and makes an action with the hand"; OBS: "Just observe"; EXE: "play the chord of your choice"

Learning by imitation: the experimental paradigm. The experiment consisted in four conditions with four events each. IMI condition (imitation): on the occurrence of the green signal, the participants had to look at the teacher's hand playing the chord (IMI-1); after a short pause (IMI-2), they have to replicate it (IMI-3). Not IMI condition: on the occurrence of the red signal (not IMI-1), the participants had to look the teacher's hand and, after a short interval (not IMI-2) touch the neck of the guitar without playing a chord (not IMI-3). OBS condition (observation): on the occurrence of the blue signal (OBS-1), the participants had to observe the neck of the guitar and, after a short pause (OBS-2), watch the teacher playing a chord (OBS-3). EXE condition (execution): on the occurrence of the yellow signal (EXE-1), the participants had to observe the neck of the guitar and, after a short interval (EXE-2) play a chord of their choice (EXE-3). In all four conditions, the experiment ended with a period in which the participants had to sit motionless (Event 4). (Buccino et al., 2004b)

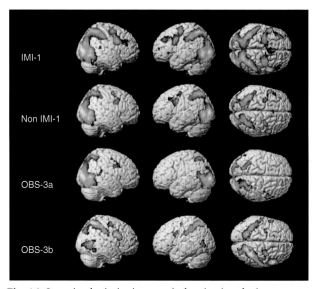

Fig. 6.2 Learning by imitation: cortical activation during observation. Cortical areas active when the participants watched the teacher playing a chord on the guitar, with the goal of imitating him (IMI-1), not with the goal of imitating him (not IMI-1), or after simply observing the neck of the guitar (OBS-3a,b). The activity in IMI-1, not IMI-1, and OBS 3a are compared with that recorded in event 4 (final pause), while OBS-3b is compared to OBS-1 (fixating the neck of the guitar). (Buccino et al., 2004b)

These data show that the transformation of visual information into an appropriate motor response takes place in the mirror neuron system; more precisely, the mirror neurons localized in the inferior parietal lobule and the frontal lobe translate the elementary acts that characterize the observed action (in this specific case, the position of the fingers required to play the chord) into motor terms.

According to Bryne's model, this condition is necessary, but not in itself sufficient, to achieve learning by imitation.

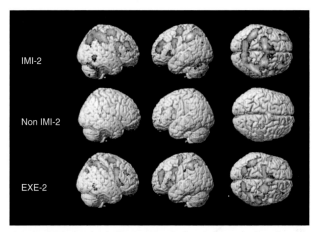

Fig. 6.3 Learning by imitation: cortical activation during the pause before execution of an action whether imitative in nature or not. All three experimental conditions were compared with Event 4 (final pause). In the IMI-2 condition the participants had to prepare to imitate the teacher, after having watched him playing a chord on the guitar; in the not IMI-2 condition, after having observed the same model as in IMI-2, they had to plan the movements of their hands (not chord playing, however) on the neck of the guitar; in EXE-2 condition they could execute a chord of their choice after having looked at the neck of the guitar. (Buccino et al., 2004b)

However the responses recorded during the intervals before imitating and before free execution of the chords, indicate that the mirror neuron system is activated under the control, so to speak, of certain areas of the frontal cortex, in particular Brodmann's area 46. In the past quite a few authors[13] have attributed area 46 with functions predominantly associated with working memory, but the results of this and other experiments suggest that there may be other functions associated

---

[13]   See for example Fuster and Alexander (1971); Funahashi *et al.* (1990).

with this area. Apart from being involved in the working memory processes, area 46 appears to be responsible for the re-combination of individual motor acts and the formation of a new pattern of action, as close as possible to that shown by the demonstrator.[14]

This analysis shows how both forms of imitation depend on the activation of the cortical areas that have mirror properties, which indicates the presence of a mechanism that matches the visual information acquired from observation of the acts of others with the corresponding motor representations. We know that in humans, as opposed to monkeys, the mirror neuron system codes both transitive and intransitive motor acts and keeps precise track of the temporal aspects of acts observed. It is therefore viable to assume that humans, with their superior motor repertoire, have a greater potential for imitation and, above all, for learning by imitation, than monkeys.

All the same, the wealth of the motor repertoire alone does not determine the capacity to learn, nor does the presence of the mirror neuron system, which is certainly a *sine qua non* condition, but not in itself *sufficient* to achieve imitation. This is true not only for the capacity to *learn* by imitation which, as we have just seen, requires the intervention of cortical areas outside the mirror neuron system, but also for the ability to *repeat* acts performed by others and belonging to our motor repertoire. Imitation requires a system which controls the mirror neurons, and this system must have two functions: facilitatory and inhibitory. It must facilitate the transition from potential action, coded by the

---

[14]   Similar interpretations are to be found in Passingham *et al.* (2000); Rowe *et al.* (2000).

mirror neurons, to the actual execution of the motor act itself when this is required by the observer; but it must also be able to inhibit this transition. If this were not so, our system would go into loop mode; every motor act we see would immediately be replicated. Fortunately for us this is not the case!

The existence of mechanisms which control the mirror neuron system is substantiated by a wealth of data, most of which is clinical. Patients with extensive lesions to the frontal lobe are known to have difficulty in stopping themselves from repeating actions they see performed by others, particularly by the doctors treating them (*imitation behaviour*). Another form of pathological behaviour may appear in patients with even more severe deficits of these control mechanisms: *echopraxia*. Patients suffering from this impairment have a compulsive tendency to imitate the acts of others immediately, even the most bizarre, almost as if it were a reflex action. So we see that lesions to the frontal lobe eliminate the braking mechanisms that block the transformation of potential actions coded by the fronto-parietal circuits into imitative acts. The block is determined by inhibition of the anterior mesial areas, such as the pre-SMA, which seem to exert an overall facilitative function over the fronto-parietal circuit.

It is probable that these mesial areas, when uninhibited following lesions of the frontal lobe, are responsible for the production of imitative acts when an individual decides that they are useful or opportune. Although there is no direct evidence of activation of these areas in the specific case of decision to imitate, electrophysiological studies have shown that the mesial cortical areas become active 800 ms before action starts, which would suggest that their activation reflects the general decision to act.

Finally, the relation between mirror mechanisms and control systems provides a clarification of certain aspects connected to precocious imitation in new-borns or pseudo-imitative behaviour in adults. An interesting observation (although sometimes contested) reveals that just a few hours after birth babies are able to reproduce certain mouth movements, such as tongue protrusion for example, that their parents make, even though they have not yet seen their own face.[15] As Andrew Meltzhoff said, 'there are no mirrors in cots!' but notwithstanding this, babies appear to be capable of this form of imitation. A possible explanation may be that they already possess a mirror neuron system, albeit rather rudimentary, and that their control mechanisms are still weak, as is also suggested by the low degree of myelinization and consequent modest functionality of the frontal lobe.

As far as adults are concerned, in 1872 Charles Darwin drew attention to certain forms of behaviour, typical of motor resonance:

> When a public singer suddenly becomes a little hoarse,
> many of those present may be heard, as I have been assured
> by a gentleman on whom I can rely, to clear their throats;
> [...]. I have also been told that at leaping matches, as the
> performer makes his spring, many of the spectators [...],
> move their feet.[16]

If we want to test the reliability of Sir Charles' statement, all we have to do is attend a football match! In any case, it is very plausible that this motor 'liberation' is due to a relaxation of the control mechanisms linked also to phenomena of emotion sharing, with the consequent appearance of

---

[15]   Meltzoff and Moore (1977).
[16]   Darwin (1872, p. 143).

movements, actions even, which would normally remain at the potential stage in the mirror neuron system.

Gestural communication

In the preceding pages we have identified a specific mechanism underlying our immediate understanding of the acts of others. This has thrown light on the neural basis of the diverse types of imitation and, as will be shown in this section, may also help in explaining the neural basis of some forms of communication, allowing us to delineate a possible scenario for the origins of human language.[17] This is not to say that the presence of a mirror neuron system, such as that found in monkeys, is sufficient to explain the emergence of intentional, or even linguistic, communicative behaviour. We have seen this when talking about imitation: it is one thing to understand an action, quite another to imitate an action we have observed. All the same, although imitation requires activation of other areas as well as those of the mirror neuron system, it would be extremely difficult for us to imitate anything at all if we did not have a mechanism to code sensory and motor information about an act or chain of acts into a common neural format. But surely this is true for any natural form of communication? Independently of whether it takes a verbal or non-verbal form, must not communication always satisfy that *parity requisite* which demands that 'the sender and the receiver must be linked by a common understanding of what counts'? How would it be possible to communicate if what is of importance for the sender were devoid of meaning for the receiver, if the 'production and perception processes' were not 'in some

---

[17]   Rizzolatti and Arbib (1998); Fogassi and Ferrari (2005).

way linked' and 'their representation' not 'at a certain point, the same'?[18]

In practical terms and independently of the neural circuits in which it is embedded, the mirror neuron system is at the root of a common space of action: if we see someone grasping food or a coffee cup in his/her hand we know immediately what they are doing. Whether that someone likes it or not, the very first signs of movement in the hand 'communicate' something to us and that something is the meaning of the act: this is what 'counts', what we share with the person who is executing the act, thanks to the activation of our motor areas. Of course, the term 'communication' is used here in the broadest sense of the word, and it certainly cannot be denied that there is an enormous gap between recognizing an act, such as grasping with the hand, and the understanding of a gesture (no matter whether it be manual, facial, or verbal) performed with an explicitly communicative intention. However, while this gap is certainly enormous, it is by no means unbridgeable.

Let us suppose, for example, that the act we are watching is of particular interest to us. In this case, when we see the other person moving their hand, our hand may tend to move in a similar manner almost without our being aware of it; this slight movement will not escape the attention of the other person and may modify their behaviour. The mirror mechanism which allowed us to understand the act of the other person from their very first movements, also ensures that we comprehend the effects our involuntary response has produced, thus creating a relationship of reciprocal interaction between our hand and that of the other person.

---

[18]   Liberman (1993); see also Liberman and Whalen (2000).

This interaction is not so very different from that 'gestural conversation' which, according to Mead, characterizes the preliminary phases of many forms of animal behaviour from fighting to courting, from caring for their young, to playing:

> There exists [...] a field of conduct even among animals below man, which in its nature may be classed as gesture. It consists of the beginnings of those actions which call out instinctive responses form other forms. These beginnings of acts call out responses which lead to readjustments of acts which have been commenced, and these readjustments lead to still other beginnings of response which again call out still other readjustments.[19]

These *mutual readjustments* endow acts performed by animals with social value, thus structuring forms of rapport that are in many ways the precursors of truly intentional communication. This latter however requires the ability to control the mirror neuron system and to incorporate the effect gestures have on the behaviour of others into motor knowledge, so that they can be recognized when seen in others. Moreover, the 'conversation' cannot just be a series of transitive gestures, it must also have access to a motor repertoire that codes intransitive, pantomimic, or expressly communicative acts.

We have already seen that many of the most common communicative gestures in monkeys, such as lip smacking or labial protrusion, have their origins in a ritualization of acts linked to ingestion (of food or of parasites removed from their partner's fur during grooming sessions), and are used to construct relationships and consolidate alliances within the tribe; also that certain mouth mirror neurons

---

[19]   Mead (1910, p. 124).

become active during ingestive acts and the observation of oro-facial communicative acts. There is a vast literature regarding arm and hand gestures in gorillas and chimpanzees that appear to have a more or less explicit communicative function, both when the animals are in the wild and when they are in captivity.[20] With regard to humans, the well-known Russian psychologist Lev Vygotskij suggested that most intransitive acts performed by children derive from transitive acts. He observed, for example, that when objects were placed within arm's reach, the children grasped them and when the objects were placed further away, they extended their arms as if to reach them. If the children's mothers responded to this tentative reaching, coming to their aid, the children repeated the gesture of reaching to indicate the objects they wished to hold.[21] On the other hand, the studies we have discussed in the preceding pages clearly show how the mirror neuron system in humans is also activated during the observation of manual pantomimes, intransitive gestures, and effective oro-facial communicative acts. Could it be possible that the progressive evolution of the mirror neuron system, whose original role was to recognize transitive manual acts such as grasping, holding, reaching, and so on, supplied the neural substrate necessary for the appearance of the first forms of communication between individuals? Could the circuit responsible for the control and production of verbal language in humans, situated in the lateral surface of the cortical hemispheres, have evolved from this system which is localized in an anatomically similar position?

---

[20] De Waal (1982); Tanner and Byrne (1996); Tomasello *et al.* (1997).
[21] Vygotskij (1934).

It can be objected that this is a rather far-fetched hypothesis, and that surely there are other, more 'economical' explanations to account for the first steps taken by humans towards language. For example, it is known that many primates emit diverse vocalizations that range from contact calls (indicating position and allowing tribes to move in a coordinated manner) to calls signalling the discovery of food or warning of the presence of predators. In a series of brilliant experiments, Dorothy Cheney and Robert Seyfarth showed how East African vervet monkeys (*Cercopithecus aethiops*) use different calls depending on whether the monkey approaching is dominant or subordinate, or on the type of action they are performing (spying on a rival tribe at a distance or moving over open territory); they also distinguish between different types of predators, using particular calls for each type (e.g. volatiles, felines, snakes, etc.) when warning tribe members of their approach.[22] Why should we not think, like Steven Pinker, that the 'first steps' in the evolution of human language were taken when a 'set of quasi-referential calls like these came under the voluntary control of the cerebral cortex', thus allowing, in the first place, the combination of a series of calls to indicate 'complicated events' and then the application of the 'ability to analyze combinations of calls [...] to the parts of each call'[23]?

There are in fact at least two good reasons to refute this evolutionary hypothesis. The *first* is functional in nature: the vocalizations of non-human primates are related exclusively

---

[22]   Cheney and Seyfarth (1990).

[23]   Pinker (1994, p. 352). It must be said that Pinker himself admitted, not without a touch of irony, that 'this idea has no more evidence in its favour than the ding-dong theory (or than Lily Tomlin's suggestion that the first human sentence was: "what a hairy back!")' (ibidem).

to emotional behaviour; moreover, even when they are semi-referential as are the calls of the vervet monkeys, they are linked to a specific function (warning, for example) and cannot be used for other purposes. In other words, the same signal cannot carry more than one message (for example 'approach' or 'escape' depending on the circumstances). Therefore these signals cannot suggest a different form of behaviour than that for which they have been generated. This does not happen in non-emotional communicative systems where the same sign can assume a multiplicity of meanings according to the context in which it is used. In human language, for example, the same word (e.g. fire), may indicate that fire has broken out ('escape' message), but it may also indicate that the fire is ready and we can prepare the meal ('approach' message). The lack of such flexibility, therefore, makes the call system of vervet monkeys unsuitable for language evolution.[24]

The *second* reason is mainly anatomic in nature: the neural circuits used by non-human primates to generate calls are radically different to those used by humans for language. The former are principally mediated by the cingulate cortex, the diencephalons, and brain stem structures[25]; the latter are localized around the lateral fissure (the fissure of Silvius) and the posterior part of the inferior frontal gyrus. Would it really be feasible to maintain that in the course of primate evolution the vocal system *bounced* from the lower regions into the lateral surface of the cortex? There is indeed a vocalization system situated in the deeper structures of the human brain, but it is linked to emotive vocal expressions such as exclamations, yells, and so on, so can hardly be considered

---

[24]   Hauser *et al.* (2002).
[25]   Juergens (2002).

as having to do with actual language. Therefore, it would surely be more logical to investigate those cortical areas in non-human primates that are homologous to those which control language in humans, focusing on the functional properties of the parieto-temporal and the inferior frontal regions.

We know that Broca's area, one of the classic areas of language, also possesses motor properties that are not exclusively verbal, becoming active during oro-facial, brachio-manual, and oro-laryngeal movements, and that its organization is similar to that found in the homologous area in monkeys, i.e. F5. Moreover Broca's area, just as F5, is a part of a mirror neuron system whose primary function is to link action understanding with action production in both humans and monkeys. This would suggest that the origins of language are to be sought, not in the primitive forms of vocal communication, but in the evolution of gestural communication controlled by the lateral cortical areas. Since the reasons given in support of the homology between Broca's area in humans and F5 in monkeys are anatomical and cytoarchitectonic—and as such are in both cases independent of the discovery of mirror neurons—the fact that there is a mechanism common to both areas (and that in humans this mechanism has new properties for the acquisition of language) seems to suggest that the progressive development of the mirror neuron system has played a key role in the appearance and evolution of the human capacity to communicate, first by gestures and later through the spoken word.

Mouth, hand, voice

The concept of the gestural origins of language is anything but new: there is the biblical-style account by etienne Bonnot de Condillac which tells the story of two children of different sex, who, after surviving the Flood, were lost in the Desert, and though totally ignorant of the 'use of signs', started to communicate by 'speaking by action'.[26] A similar view can be found in the psychological considerations penned by Wilhelm Wundt on the 'natural course' of a language of gestures, which, though 'imperfect', and mostly linked to 'mimetic representations', produced an early 'form of discourse', which was only later integrated with phonetics.[27] However the most important support for this view has emerged over the last two decades, drawing on palaeontology, ethology, neurophysiology, and comparative anatomy; it has acquired numerous supporters, especially among those who sustain the so-called sensory–motor theories of language production and perception.[28]

Take, for example, Peter MacNeilage: this author maintains that the mouth open–close alternation would provide the 'syllabic frame' typical of human language while its modulation would determine the various 'contents' (vowels and consonants). This mouth open–close alternation would represent the evolutionary outcome of the articulatory system, which originated from the mandibular cycle typical of chewing and ingesting food. In his view, this would be supported by the fact that in non-human primates most of the cortical changes necessary for the emergence of language have taken place in the frontal region, which is the homologue to Broca's area and fundamentally controls mastication.[29]

---

[26] Condillac (1746, pp. 175–176).
[27] Wundt (1916, p. 128).
[28] See, for example, Armstrong *et al.* (1995); Armstrong (1999); Corballis (1992; 2002; 2003).
[29] MacNeilage (1998).

The discovery of mouth mirror neurons in the ventral premotor cortex in the monkey seems to support MacNeilage's theory, which, however, appears to underestimate the role of brachio-manual gestures in language evolution. It is in fact the anatomical and functional architecture of F5 and Broca's area, both characterized by brachio-manual motor representations (and not only by oro-facial and oro-laryngeal ones), that suggests that inter-individual communication did not evolve from a single motor modality but from the progressive integration of facial, brachio-manual, and, last but not least, vocal gestures accompanied, as we will see later, by the appearance of the relative mirror neuron systems. Paraphrasing Michael Corballis, it can be said that the origins of language are not to be found in the mouth alone, but also in the hand, and their mutual interaction gave origin to speech.[30] It cannot be denied that the potential of communication would be extremely limited without a brachio-manual system in support of the oro-facial. Reflect for a while on the importance of the hand in communication; it permits us to introduce a 'third party' into person-to-person communication by indicating the position of a third individual or an object and describing certain of their characteristics. The first open communication system that expressed new meanings by exploiting the possible combinations of individual movements (which does not happen in the oro-facial communications of primates) certainly owes more to the use of the hand than to the use of the mouth.

As pointed out recently by Michael Arbib, the ability of the hominids first to imitate, then to mime the acts of their motor repertoire, and finally to perform brachio-manual

---

[30]   Corballis (2002, p. 153).

'proto-signs' to render their communications precise and reliable, must have played a decisive role in the evolution of this communication system.[31] This inevitably resulted in radical transformations at the cerebral level, especially in the motor cortex. It is likely that our non-human ancestors of 20 million years ago possessed a mirror neuron system that allowed the execution and recognition of simple motor acts such as grasping, holding, and so on, and that the ancestor that we share with chimpanzees, 5 or 6 million years ago, also had mirror neurons that enabled it to perform rudimentary forms of imitation. Unfortunately only a few fossils remain from the period between the time of the human–chimpanzee split and the appearance of the first australopithecines, but analyses done on traces of cerebral circumvolutions in the cavities of a number of *Homo habilis* skulls, dating back almost 2 million years, show that the frontal and temporo-parietal regions were strongly developed at that stage in the evolution process.[32] This suggests that the transition from australopithecines to *Homo habilis* coincided with the transition to a more differentiated mirror system, which supplied the neural substrate for the formation of the 'mimic culture' which, according to Merlin Donald, peaked with the appearance on the scene of *Homo erectus*, who walked the earth from 1.5 million to 300 thousand years ago.[33] It is also plausible to suppose that mirror neurons evolved further during the transition, 250 thousand years ago, from *Homo erectus* to *Homo sapiens*, responding to the expansion both of the motor repertoire and the newly acquired ability to communicate intentionally by

---

[31]   Arbib (2002;2005).
[32]   Tobias (1987); Holloway (1983;1985); Falk (1983).
[33]   Donald (1991).

manual gestures that gradually became more articulate and was frequently accompanied by vocalizations.

It is probable that the development of the brachio-manual communication system modified the importance of vocalizations and above all of how they were controlled. This is not to say that they were not present during oro-facial communications, quite the contrary. However in this case the addition of sound to the communication had an emotive significance and served to reinforce the message ('anger' or 'joy' for example). They did not require any precise form of execution, and this explains why this kind of vocalization remained under the control of the old system that was localized predominantly in the sub-cortical centres. This must have changed radically when sounds were used together with mimic and manual 'proto-signs' in intentional communications: as had happened with hand gestures previously, precision, descriptive capacity, expressive relia-bility were now required for vocalizations, as was the ability to recognize these skills and learn them by imitation. If this had not been possible, it is unlikely that vocal communica-tion could have functioned in parallel with gestural communication to finally usurp its importance. However this also required the recruitment of new cortical areas to control the emission of sounds—and this could probably be the origin of the modern Broca's area, equipped with mirror properties, representation of oro-laryngeal movements, and in addition, a very close link with the adjacent primary motor cortex.

In the early 1930s Sir Richard Paget attempted to dem-onstrate how vocal 'proto-signs', like their manual counter-parts, were linked to mimic, and that this enabled them to assume a communicative function, thus resulting in a verbal 'proto-language' with a somewhat primitive vocabulary and extremely rudimentary syntax.[34] By analysing the roots of a number of words from very different languages ranging from Polynesian and Chinese to some Semitic and Indo-European languages, Paget discovered a certain parallelism between sounds and meaning, which, in his opinion, was due to the fact that the movements of the mouth, lips, and especially of the tongue reproduced in miniature mimes executed by the hands and other parts of the body and were accompanied by specific sound emissions. Not only was this connection between gestures and sound conserved in the course of evolution, it also marked the beginning of spoken language as such. He maintained, for example, that the use of vowels such as 'A' and 'I' depended not so much on the quality of the sound, but was dictated by reference to something large or small respectively, as the form the mouth assumes when emitting these sounds reproduces the shape assumed by the hands to grasp the object. The same is true for other sounds such as 'M' for example, which indicates a permanent state of closure or 'TR', which denotes running or walking.

Of course this is just a speculative hypothesis, sometimes based on unproved considerations, but it is less ingenuous than was thought for many years, as is now recognized, among others, by the American linguist Morris Swadesh.[35] Be that as it may, this theory makes a valid effort to explain how a visually transparent system, such as the brachio-manual system, was integrated and later supplanted by an opaque system such as oro-laryngeal gestures, without losing the capacity to transmit meaning and therefore to communicate. Moreover, from the neurophysiologic point

---

[34]   Paget (1930). See Bickerton (1995) for the notion of proto-language.
[35]   Swadesh (1972).

of view, this would mean that the two gestural systems are closely linked at cortical level, based on a partly common neural substrate—and a number of recent studies have shown that this would appear to be the case.

TMS experiments, in fact, show how the excitability of right hand motor representation increases during reading or speaking.[36] The effect is limited to the representation of the right hand and does not include the motor area of the leg. It must be noted that the excitability of the motor cortex of the hand could not be ascribed to verbal articulation, as this is a function common to both hemispheres, while the increase observed occurred in the left hemisphere only. It therefore follows that the recorded facilitation must have been caused by the co-activation of the motor area of the right hand and the language circuit.

Maurizio Gentilucci and colleagues[37] arrived at a similar conclusion using an entirely different approach. They asked the participants in their experiment to grasp two objects of differing size with their mouths while opening their right hands at the same time. Their results showed that the widest finger span was obtained when the participants opened their mouths for the larger of the two objects. Even more pertinent to demonstrating the close connection between manual acts and oro-laryngeal gestures is their experiment in which the participants were shown two three-dimensional objects, one large and one small, with two symbols or series of marks on the visible surface. The participants were asked to grasp the objects, but when the symbols were visible they had also to open their mouths. The recordings of the

[36]   Meister *et al.* (2003); see also Tokimura *et al.* (1996); Seyal *et al.* (1999).
[37]   Gentilucci *et al.* (2001).

kinematics of the hand, arm, and mouth showed that in spite of the fact that the participants had been instructed to open their mouths in the same way in all the experimental conditions, they opened their mouths wider when the hand movement was directed to the larger of the two objects. Control experiments clearly showed that the effect was specific for the movements of the mouth and the contralateral hand, and that simultaneous extension of the contralateral forearm in no way influenced the execution of the task.

These authors also conducted another experiment using the same set-up as before, but asking the participants to pronounce a syllable (such as GU or GA) instead of simply opening their mouths. The syllables were marked on the objects in the same position as the symbols in the previous experiment. They found that the maximum lip aperture and vocal spectrum power during syllable emission occured when the participants were grasping the larger object.

As shown above, both the simple movements of the mouth and the oro-laryngeal synergies required for syllable production are linked to manual gestures; moreover motor acts requiring a large aperture of the hand and oro-laryngeal acts requiring a large aperture of the mouth appear to be based on a common neural organization that represents a *vestigia* of the stage in the evolution of language in which sound started to convey meaning thanks to the capacity of the mouth and oro-laryngeal systems to articulate gestures with a semantic value analogous to those coded by the manual system.

Gentilucci and his colleagues also showed that grasping hand movements influence syllable pronunciation even when they are not being carried out in the first person, but being observed. In another experiment, the participants were asked to pronounce the syllables BA or GA while watching another person picking up objects of varying sizes.[38] Kinematics of lip aperture and spectrum of voice amplitude were influenced by the grasping movements of the other person; specifically, both lip aperture and voice peak amplitude were greater when the observed action was directed at larger objects. It is worth noting at this point that the existence of a link between gestural and vocal systems is confirmed by a number of clinical studies. For example, it has been observed that pointing to objects on a screen with the right hand facilitates aphasics in naming tasks[39], and similarly that the use of manual gestures can help patients with cerebral lesions to recover the use of speech.[40]

But let us return, briefly, to the evolutionary scenario. It is very probable that evolutionary pressure to produce more complex forms of communication boosted the development of a highly sophisticated neural control mechanism for phonation, which would then have controlled not only specific sound emission, but also created an increasingly wider (indeed, potentially infinite) group of possible combinations that eventually caused the vocal system to split from the gestural. How and when the vocal system acquired full autonomy, relegating the gestural system to the status of an accessory factor to sound communication, is still a matter of debate. It could well be a quite recent event, linked to the appearance of the vocal tract typical of *Homo sapiens*[41], although some authors have proffered alternative solutions.[42] In any case, it is reasonable to suppose that this process (or another similar) was accompanied by radical cortical

---

[38] Gentilucci (2003).
[39] Hanlon *et al.* (1990).
[40] Hadar *et al.* (1998).
[41] Lieberman (1975).
[42] See, for example, Gibson and Jessee (1999).

transformations, regarding in particular the motor centres assigned to the production and reception of verbal material. However, these transformations would have been totally useless without the contemporaneous evolution of the mechanism that was able to satisfy what we have seen to be the *sine qua non* condition for any form of communication, in other words, the *parity condition* that ensures the *sender and the receiver share an understanding of what counts.*

Alvin Liberman, who more than any other researcher investigated the conditions necessary for any communicative conduct, showed that in linguistic communication it is not the sounds that count, but the articulatory gestures by which these are generated because the latter provide the former with phonetic consistence. This is how we are able immediately to perceive the difference between the syllable BA and a cough.[43] If we accept his interpretation (and much of the evidence he adduced in over thirty years of research would support this line of thought), we must recognize that the transition to an autonomous vocal system must have meant that the motor neurons responsible for controlling the oro-laryngeal gestures acquired the capacity to become active in response to sounds produced by similar gestures by others; in other words, the mirror neuron system underwent a further reorganization in order to guarantee the transformation of verbal sounds into motor representations of corresponding articulatory gestures. The discovery of a new mirror neuron system, the *echo-mirror neuron system*, constitutes evidence that this reorganization did actually happen.[44]

An experiment conducted by Luciano Fadiga and his colleagues provided the first indication of the existence of

---

[43]   Liberman and Whalen (2000).
[44]   Rizzolatti and Buccino (2005).

this mirror neuron system. They asked their participants to listen carefully to verbal and non-verbal stimuli (words, regular pseudo-words, and bitonal sounds), while the experimenters recorded MEPs from their tongue muscles during this activity. A double 'F' or a double 'R' was embedded in the words and the pseudo-words. 'F' is a labio-dental fricative that, when pronounced, requires only slight movement of the tongue, whereas 'R' is a linguo-palatal fricative that involves a marked movement of the tongue. The experimenters noted that when the participants heard words or pseudo-words containing a double 'R', there was a significant increase in the MEPs recorded from the tongue muscles compared to when they listened to bitonal sounds, words, and pseudo-words containing a double 'F' (Figure 6.4).[45]

Tomáš M. Paus and colleagues[46] obtained similar results from a TMS experiment recording MEPs from the lips (the *orbicularis oris* muscle) in four conditions: listening to continuous prose, to non-verbal sounds, viewing lip movements during speech, and viewing movements of the eyes and eyebrows. When the participants listened to speech or viewed speech movements, there was an increase in the MEPs recorded from the *orbicularis oris* muscle, but only in response to stimulation of the left hemisphere. In fact, stimulation of the right hemisphere did not result in any modification to the MEPs in any of the experimental conditions.

All in all, the neurophysiological data obtained from these experiments, and those described previously, indicate that the long process of evolution towards language has been marked by a series of important events (the integration of the oro-facial and manual systems, the formation of

---

[45]   Fadiga *et al.* (2002).
[46]   Watkins *et al.* (2003).

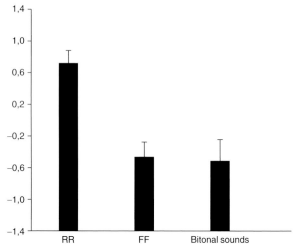

Fig. 6.4 Motor evoked potentials (MEPs) recorded from the tongue muscles while listening to verbal material and bitonal sounds. The graph shows the data of all the participants. RR refers to the verbal stimuli containing linguo-palatal fricatives, FF to the verbal material containing labio-dental fricatives. (Modified from Fadiga et al., 2002)

a repertoire of predominantly mimetic gestural 'proto-signs', the emergence of a bimodal 'proto-language' formed of gestures and sounds, and finally the appearance of a prevalently vocal system of communication), each of which appears to be linked to a phase in the development of a mechanism, such as that of the mirror neurons, that was originally assigned to recognizing the actions of others and devoid of any effective intentional communicative function. Of course, this is just one of the many possible scenarios: given the extreme complexity of the factors that contribute to determining the capacity of language, much new research is necessary. All the same, we are convinced that the study of the properties of mirror neurons and the various systems in which they are involved, allows the individuation of some of the neural structures which, once again in Pinker's words, 'would have given evolution some parts it could think with to produce the human language circuitry'.[47]

[47]   Pinker (1994, p. 350).

CHAPTER 7

Sharing emotions

The role of emotions

In the preceding chapters we have considered actions carried out or perceived in contexts devoid of emotional content—a choice essentially dictated by methodological reasons, as only emotionally neutral experimental conditions are suitable to determine the specific components of actions within the intricate architecture of motor phenomena. Had a different approach been adopted, it would have been difficult to identify the mechanisms and cortical circuits of the sensory motor transformations responsible for the codification of objects, the planning and control of our actions, and the understanding of the actions and intentions of others. However, emotions are an integral part of our life; they allow us to immediately assess variations in our surroundings, whether expected or not, and react to them to our best advantage.

Things are hardly ever just within reach or out of reach, graspable or not graspable, graspable with the hand or mouth, with this or that grip: they almost always incorporate a threat or an opportunity, are repulsive or attractive, provoke fear or wonder, disgust or interest, pain or pleasure, and so on.

The same applies to the people we meet: their behaviour not only embodies particular acts, but often provokes in us feelings of anger, hate, terror, admiration, compassion, hope, and so on. Irrespective of whether we are aware of these feelings or not, or whether they produce an effect which is explicit and recognizable by others, or simply create internal physiological reactions, our emotions supply our brain with an important instrument for navigating the sea of sensory information and automatically triggering the most appropriate responses to ensure our survival and well being. True, they sometimes deceive us: who can honestly say that they have never panicked for no good reason? All the same, if we were not able to feel fear, or, in more general terms, if our brain were not able to discriminate at emotional level events perceived, remembered, or imagined, it would be almost impossible for us to deal with even the most banal of the situations that we have to face daily.

In his 1872 masterpiece, *The Expression of the Emotions*, Darwin taught us that most of our emotive reactions, and in particular those known as the primary emotions (fear, anger, disgust, pain, surprise, joy, and so on), consist in a collection of responses that have been conserved during the course of evolution due to their original adaptive utility; he points out that it is not surprising they occur in the same form in different species and, in humans, in different cultures. Take pain, for example:

> When animals suffer from an agony of pain, they generally writhe about with frightful contortions; and those which habitually use their voices utter piercing cries or groans. Almost every muscle of the body is brought into strong action. With man the mouth may be closely compressed, or more commonly the lips are retracted, with the teeth clenched or ground together. There is said to be 'gnashing of teeth' in hell; and I have plainly heard the grinding of the molar teeth of a cow which was suffering acutely from inflammation of the bowels.

The female hippopotamus in the Zoological Gardens, when she produced her young, suffered greatly; she incessantly walked about, or rolled on her sides, opening and closing her jaws, and clattering her teeth together. With man the eyes stare wildly as in horrified astonishment, or the brows are heavily contracted. Perspiration bathes the body, and drops trickle down the face. The circulation and respiration are much affected. Hence the nostrils are generally dilated and often quiver; or the breath may be held until the blood stagnates in the purple face. If the agony be severe and prolonged, these signs all change; utter prostration follows, with fainting or convulsions.[1]

Or think of the disgust we feel when seeing or tasting food to which we are not accustomed:

In Tierra del Fuego a native touched with his finger some cold preserved meat which I was eating at our bivouac, and plainly showed utter disgust at its softness; whilst I felt utter disgust at my food being touched by a naked savage, though his hands did not appear dirty. A smear of soup on a man's beard looks disgusting, though there is of course nothing disgusting in the soup itself. I presume that this follows from the strong association in our minds between the sight of food, however circumstanced, and the idea of eating it. As the sensation of disgust primarily arises in connection with the act of eating or tasting, it is natural that its expression should consist chiefly in movements round the mouth. But as disgust also causes annoyance, it is generally accompanied by a frown, and often by gestures as if to push away or to guard oneself against the offensive object. [...] With respect to the face, moderate disgust is exhibited in various ways; by the mouth being widely opened, as if to let an offensive morsel drop out; by spitting; by blowing out of the protruded lips; or by a sound as of clearing the throat. [...] Extreme disgust is expressed by movements round the mouth identical with those preparatory to the act of vomiting.

---

[1]   Darwin (1872, p. 70).

The mouth is opened widely, with the upper lip strongly retracted, which wrinkles the sides of the nose, and with the lower lip protruded and everted as much as possible. This latter movement requires the contraction of the muscles which draw downwards the corners of the mouth. It is remarkable how readily and instantly retching or actual vomiting is induced in some persons by the mere idea of having partaken of any unusual food, as of an animal which is not commonly eaten; although there is nothing in such food to cause the stomach to reject it. When vomiting results, as a reflex action, from some real cause—as from too rich food, or tainted meat, or from an emetic—it does not ensue immediately, but generally after a considerable interval of time. Therefore, to account for retching or vomiting being so quickly and easily excited by a mere idea, the suspicion arises that our progenitors must formerly have had the power (like that possessed by ruminants and some other animals) of voluntarily rejecting food which disagreed with them, or which they thought would disagree with them; and now, though this power has been lost, as far as the will is concerned, it is called into involuntary action, through the force of a formerly well-established habit, whenever the mind revolts at the idea of having partaken of any kind of food, or at anything disgusting.[2]

We are now beginning to have a fair knowledge of the anatomy and function of the principal nervous centres that are responsible for the primary emotions such as pain and disgust as well as the role these centres play in the organization of cerebral activity and regulation of the vital processes. However the study of the neurophysiological bases of the emotions is not limited to the mechanisms by which the brain picks up danger signals or traces of nauseating tastes or smells, and triggers the routing of adaptive responses so clearly described by Darwin. Most of our interactions with

---

[2]   Darwin (1872, pp. 257–259).

the environment and our emotive conduct depend on our capacity to perceive and understand the emotions of others. We are concerned when we see a person turn pale and start to tremble: if we see him running away, this constitutes a powerful emotive stimulus for us, much more powerful than if we see him merely walking away. The same is true if we see a grimace of disgust on the face of someone eating; it is most unlikely that we will rush to secure a piece of the same food for ourselves.

There are obvious advantages in these forms of emotive behaviour. Not only do they ensure that the single individuals are able to effectively deal with threats and opportunities, they also enable the creation and consolidation of the first inter-individual bonding. We know that as early as the second and third days of life babies are able to distinguish between happy and sad faces[3] and that by their second or third month they develop an affective consonance with their mother, to the extent that they reproduce more or less synchronized facial expressions and/or vocalizations that reflect her emotive state.[4] The articulation and progressive differentiation of the emotive awakening induced by the perception of the expressions of those around them, allow babies to formulate basic social skills in the following months such as offering help and comfort.[5] These are mostly rudimentary forms of empathy, much less sophisticated than those underlying our social conduct when we reach maturity, but both require the capacity to understand the emotions of others, to read signs of pain, fear, disgust, and joy in their faces and body language.

---

[3] Field *et al.* (1982).
[4] Stern (1995).
[5] Bretherton *et al.* (1986); Zahn-Waxler *et al.* (1992).

What mechanism does our brain use to process stimuli from, say, a particular facial expression, and code it as *a grimace of pain* or *disgust*? Must we assume that the activation of the visual cortical areas triggers cognitive processes that will allow us to interpret sensory information as laden with a particular emotive significance? Or should we rather suppose that the sight of an emotion on the face of another will activate in the observer those same cerebral centres that become active when he experiences that same emotion? In other words, does the understanding of the emotions of others rest on a complex of neural circuits that, though different to those seen in action understanding, also have mirror properties? Or is it a cognitive process which basically does not differ from that underlying the visual recognition of faces or more generally of shapes, except for the type of processed information?

Disgusted together in the Island of Reil?

Let us take a closer look at disgust. In its primitive manifestation, this primary emotion is linked to the ingestion, tasting, and smelling of food and is characterized by mouth and labial movements, a wrinkling of the nose, and, in extreme forms, by nausea and retching.[6] In recent years a number of experimental studies have individuated the cerebral areas that are principally involved in reactions of disgust to gustatory and olfactory stimuli, ascertaining that the key role is played by the cortical area known as the insular lobe or *insula of Reil* (Figure 7.1).

---

[6] For a recent classification of typical reactions of disgust, see Rozin *et al.* (2000).

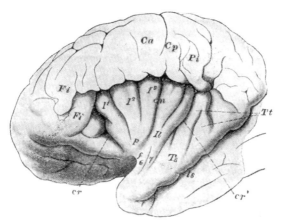

Fig. 7.1 The insular lobe, or insula, is situated in the depths of the lateral fossa (known also as the fissure of Silvius). In the diagram it is exposed by slightly parting the opercula of the lateral fossa and turning down the temporal lobe. (Chiarugi, 1954.)

It has long been known that the insula is not a homogeneous structure. In the monkey, for example, it is generally subdivided into three cytoarchitectonic areas: the agranular, dysgranular, and granular insula. If however we turn our attention to its connections with the cerebral cortex and the subcortical centres, we see that it can be subdivided into two major sectors with different functional properties: an anterior, 'visceral' region that coincides with the agranular insula and the anterior part of the dysgranular insula, and a polymodal posterior region that includes the posterior part of the dysgranular and the granular insula.[7] The anterior region is closely connected with the gustatory and

---

[7] See Mesulam and Mufson (1982a,b); Mufson and Mesulam (1982).

olfactory centres[8]; in addition it receives information from the anterior region of the ventral part of the superior temporal sulcus (STS), where there are many neurons that respond to the sight of faces.[9] The posterior region, on the other hand, characterized by its connections with the auditory, somatosensory, and premotor cortical areas, is not directly linked to the gustatory or olfactory centres.

Recently it was discovered that the insula represents the primary cortical area not only for chemical *exteroception* (smell and taste) but also for *enteroception*, i.e. the reception of signals relative to the interior body states. These signals ascend the spinal chord and reach specific sectors of the thalamus, which, in turn, project topographically to the various sectors of the insula.[10] This is all the more interesting if we keep in mind that the insula, particularly its anterior region, is a visceromotor integration centre: when it is stimulated electrically, it causes a series of bodily movements that, unlike those induced by the stimulation of motor areas, are accompanied by visceral effects such as an increase in heart beat, dilation of the pupils, retching, and similar sensations.[11]

The human insula is much larger than that of the monkey, but its architecture is very similar.[12] In agreement with the anatomical data just reviewed[13], brain imaging studies have shown that the anterior part of the insula becomes active in response to gustatory and olfactory stimuli (and with regards the latter the activations are stronger in the left hemisphere

---

[8]   Yaxley *et al.* (1990); Scott *et al.* (1991); Augustine (1996).
[9]   Bruce *et al.* (1981); Perrett *et al.* (1982;1984;1985); Desimone *et al.* (1984).
[10] Craig (2002).
[11] Kaada *et al.* (1949); Frontera (1956); Showers and Lauer (1961).
[12] Mesulam and Mufson (1982a).
[13] Zald *et al.* (1998a); Zald and Pardo (2000); Royet *et al.* (2003).

than in the right).[14] Furthermore, as in the monkey, stimulation of the insula carried out on neurosurgical patients often provokes visceromotor reactions such as nausea, retching and unpleasant, sometimes intolerable, sensations in the throat and mouth.[15]

Another very important finding is that the anterior region of the insula is activated by facial expressions of disgust seen on the faces of others.[16] Mary Phillips and colleagues found that the intensity of the activation of the insular cortex is proportional to the degree of disgust observed.[17] Their results were corroborated by Pierre Krolak-Salmon and colleagues, who, recording evoked potentials from the insula of epileptic patients for diagnostic purposes, observed that the anterior region of the insula responded selectively to the sight of disgusted faces.[18] In addition recent clinical studies have provided further demonstrations of the importance of the activation of the insular cortex not only for triggering sensations and reactions of disgust, but also for perceiving this emotion on the face of others.

Andrew J. Calder and colleagues[19] reported the case of a patient (NK) who, following a cerebral haemorrhage, had severe damage to the left insula and its surrounding structures. He was no longer able to recognize visual expressions of aversion, although his visual perception of other emotions was not affected. Not only was his ability to perceive disgust

---

[14] Royet *et al.* (2000; 2001; 2003); Zald and Pardo (1997); Zald *et al.* (1998b); Zald (2003).

[15] Penfield and Faulk (1955); Krolak-Salmon *et al.* (2003).

[16] Phillips *et al.* (1997;1998); Sprengelmeyer *et al.* (1998); Schienle *et al.* (2002).

[17] Phillips *et al.* (1997).

[18] Krolak-Salmon *et al.* (2003).

[19] Calder *et al.* (2000).

impaired visually, but also acoustically: the sound of retching, for example, had no emotive meaning for him, though laughter and other emotive reactions did. This polymodal deficit also affected his personal experiences: in fact, NK maintained that while he was able to feel fear or anger, he experienced only vague feelings of revulsion.

Ralph Adolphs and colleagues[20] studied a similar case. The insula of their patient (B) had extensive bilateral lesions. Like NK, he was no longer able to identify facial expressions of disgust. To verify the polymodality of his deficit, B was presented with a series of situations that typically produce a reaction of disgust, such as the ingestion, regurgitation, and spitting out of food, accompanied by noisy retching and grimaces. B did not show any sign of being disgusted maintaining, on the contrary, that the food was 'delicious'. His inability to experience disgust was confirmed by the fact that he no longer discriminated what he ate, swallowing things that were totally inedible, and showing no reaction to food stimuli which were disgusting to others.

We have seen that clinical data as well as brain imaging and electrostimulation studies seem to indicate that experiencing disgust and perceiving it in others have a common neural substrate and that the involvement of the insula is fundamental in both cases. This would appear to suggest that the real understanding of disgust experienced by others, i.e. when the observer effectively understands what the other person is experiencing in a given moment, does not assume nor is it based on inferential or associative cognitive processes. However, more direct evidence is needed to substantiate the existence of a mirror mechanism

---

[20]   Adolphs *et al.* (2003).

and to guarantee that the *same region* of the insula becomes active both when we experience revulsion ourselves and when we see it expressed by others.

This was the objective of the study conducted by Bruno Wicker and colleagues[21], in which healthy volunteers were subjected to an fMRI experiment subdivided in two different sessions. In the first session, which dealt with the olfactory aspect of the issue, the participants were exposed to both disgusting and pleasant odours; in the second session, devoted to the visual aspect of the issue, they were asked to watch people in a video sniffing three odours, one disgusting, one pleasant, and one neutral, to which they reacted with a grimace, a look of pleasure, or indifference respectively (Figure 7.2).

Two of the structures that became active during the exposure to smell were of great interest: the amygdala and the insula. Both disgusting and pleasant odours activated the amygdala (a subcortical structure that mediates various emotional responses), with a clear overlap of the regions they activated (Figure 7.3A).

Conversely, the disgusting smells activated the anterior region of the right and left insula, while the pleasant odours activated a more posterior site in the right insula only (Figure 7.3B).

In the visual session, only the sight of the grimace of disgust activated the insula. The most important finding here was that this activation coincided in the anterior part of the left insula with that which occured when the participants sniffed the disgusting smells (Figure 7.4).

There was also a certain degree of overlapping of the areas activated by disgusting smells and the sight of faces

---

[21]   Wicker *et al.* (2003).

Disgust   Pleasure   Neutral

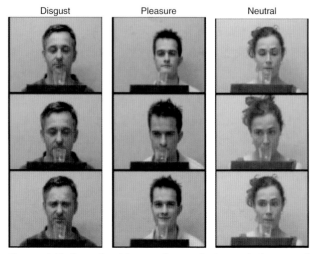

Fig. 7.2 Stills from the videos used to study the cortical areas and the subcortical centres activated while observing faces expressing emotions. The demonstrators sniffed a glass containing pure water or water mixed with unpleasant and pleasant smells. The faces of the demonstrators expressed disgust, pleasure or indifference depending on the stimulus. The experiment used six demonstrators, each of whom sniffed the contents of the glass in the three conditions (Wicker et al., 2003.)

expressing disgust in the anterior part of the right cingulated cortex. Conversely, there was no activation in the amygdala while observing disgusted faces, which concurred with the findings of some previous studies that showed dissociation between the neural circuits underlying recognition of fear, in which the amygdala is strongly involved, and those underlying disgust, in which it would not appear to have a particularly important role to play.[22]

---

[22]   See for example, Calder *et al.* (2001).

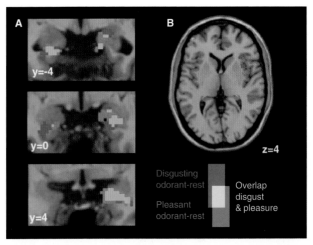

Fig. 7.3 Activations during olfactory stimulation. The activations are superimposed on the anatomical image of a standard brain (MNI – Montreal Neurological Institute), adopting neurological conventions (right is right). (A) Coronal sections through the amygdalae. Note the vast area of overlapping (shaded in yellow) of the activations triggered by the unpleasant (red) and pleasant (green) smells in the right amygdala. (B) Horizontal section showing activations in the insula. The activation for the unpleasant smells is bilateral and anterior, while it is more posterior and limited to the right hemisphere for the pleasant smells. There is no overlapping for the two types of odour. (Wicker et al., 2003.)

Empathy and emotive colouring

Experiencing disgust and perceiving it in others appear therefore to have a common neural base, constituted by the anterior region of the left insula and the cingulate cortex of the right hemisphere. The overlapping of the cerebral activations found following the inhalation of disgusting smells and during observation of expressions of disgust on the faces of other people confirms the hypothesis that the

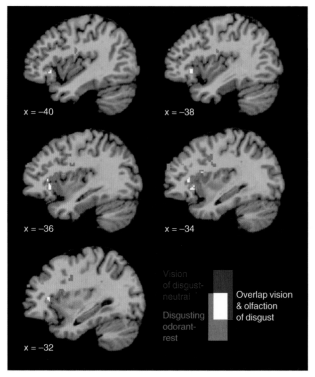

Fig. 7.4 Activations during olfactory stimulation with unpleasant smells and during the sight of faces grimacing in disgust. The blue areas indicate the activations triggered by the faces expressing disgust, the red areas those triggered by unpleasant smells and the white areas the sites activated by both types of stimuli. The activations are shown on a sagittal section of a standard brain (MNI–Montreal Neurological Institute). (Wicker et al., 2003.)

understanding of the emotive states of others depends on a mirror mechanism that codes the sensory information directly in emotional terms. The visual stimulus autonomously and selectively activated the same areas involved in the emotional response to the olfactory experience, thus enabling immediate understanding of the meaning of a facial grimace, distinguishing it without difficulty from other emotive expressions. The cases of NK and B clearly showed how their incapacity to understand the reactions of others was closely linked to their inability to experience the emotions themselves.

What we have just expounded appears to be valid for all the primary emotions and not just disgust. Take pain, for example. Some years ago William D. Hutchison and his colleagues[23] recorded the activity of single neurons in patients who had to undergo a partial ablation of the cingulate cortex for therapeutic reasons. They found that there are neurons in the anterior part of this cortex that respond both to the application of a painful stimulus to the patient's hand and when the patient watches this stimulus being applied to the hands of others.

More recently Tania Singer and co-workers[24] conducted an fMRI experiment in which the participants were subjected to a painful electric shock from electrodes placed on their hand, while in another condition they were asked to watch while the same electrodes were fastened to the hand of a person to whom they were deeply attached sentimentally. They were told that this person would receive the same electric shocks to which they had been subjected earlier. In both conditions, sectors of the anterior insula and the cingulate cortex became active, showing that both direct suffering and its evocation are mediated by a mirror mechanism similar to that demonstrated for disgust.

It is worth nothing that the interpretation of emotion understanding presented here is not very different to that

---

[23]   Hutchison *et al.* (1999).

[24]   Singer *et al.* (2004).

proposed by Antonio Damasio and his co-workers[25], although it does diverge on one aspect. In Damasio's view, it is the areas of the somatosensory cortex and the insula that are involved in experiencing an emotion and recognizing it in others. The sight of disgust or pain on the face of another person would produce a modification in the activation of the observer's corporeal maps, so that he would perceive the emotion of the other person 'as if' it were his own.

> The presumed mechanism for producing this sort of feeling is a variety of what I have called the 'as-if-body-loop' mechanism. It involves an internal brain simulation that consists of a rapid modification of ongoing body maps. This is achieved when certain brain regions, such as the prefrontal/premotor cortices, directly signal the body-sensing brain regions. The existence and location of comparable types of neurons has been established recently. Those neurons can represent, in individual's brain, the movement that very brain sees in another individual, and produce signals toward sensorimotor structures so that the corresponding movements are either 'previewed', in simulation mode, or actually executed.[26]

In other words, observation of the faces of others expressing an emotion would activate the mirror neurons of the premotor cortex. These neurons would then send a copy of their activation pattern (*an efferent copy*) to the somatosensory areas and the insula. The activation of these areas, analogous to what occurs when the observer spontaneously expresses that emotion ('as if'), would be at the root of our understanding of the emotive reactions of others.

Now there is no doubt that our motor system mirrors the facial movements of others, but, as we have seen, this is also

---

[25]   See for example, Damasio (2003); Adolphs (2001; 2002; 2003).
[26]   Damasio (2003, pp. 115–116).

true when these movements have no emotive significance. In our opinion it is pleonastic to assume involvement of the sensory cortex areas in recognizing the emotions of others (Damasio himself admits this when he indicates the insula as being the most important region of the 'as if' circuit)[27]. The information from the visual areas, providing descriptions of faces or bodies expressing emotion, is conveyed directly to the insula, where it autonomously and specifically activates a mirror mechanism that immediately codes these descriptions in the corresponding emotive mode. The insula is the centre of this mirror system, not only because it is the cortical region in which the internal states of the body are represented, but because it is the visceromotor integration centre, which, when activated, provokes the transformation of sensory input into visceral reactions.

The experiments conducted by Wicker *et al.* and Singer *et al.*, as well as the stimulation studies that we have described earlier, show how these visceral reactions qualify the emotive responses of the patients and the participants, as well as their perception of the emotive responses of others[28]. This does not mean that we would not be able to discriminate the emotions of others without the insula, but to quote William James, our perception of these would be reduced to a perception 'purely cognitive in form, pale, colourless, destitute of emotional warmth'[29]. Therefore the 'emotional warmth', i.e. the emotive colouring, would depend on the sharing of the visceromotor responses that contribute to define the actual emotions.

It is well known that the sight of someone retching induces a similar reaction in the observer, who maybe will

[27] Damasio (2003, p. 133).
[28] Damasio (2003, p. 145).
[29] James (1890, p. 450).

not actually vomit, but will almost certainly experience a sense of nausea, cramps in the stomach, etc., just as if he had eaten or imbibed something particularly disgusting. The fact that the visceromotor reactions provoked by the activation of the insula do not necessarily have an effect on the peripheral centres does not mean that they are totally irrelevant. Quite the contrary, they represent a potential visceromotor activity that may be either executed or remain at the potential state, but in both cases it is indispensable for a first person understanding the emotions of others.

We do not need to reproduce the behaviour of others in full detail in order to understand its emotive meaning, just as action understanding does not require the actions to be replicated. Even if they involve different cortical circuits, our perceptions of the motor acts and emotive reactions of others appear to be united by a mirror mechanism that permits our brain to immediately understand what we are seeing, feeling, or imagining others to be doing, as it triggers the same neural structures (motor or visceromotor respectively) that are responsible for our own actions and emotions. We have already mentioned that this mirror mechanism is not the only way our brain has of understanding the acts and intentions of others and this is true also for emotions: they may be understood by means of a reflexive processing of the sensory aspects linked to how they appear in the facial expressions or acts of others. It is important to remember however that this processing alone, without the support of a visceromotor mirroring, will remain that 'colourless' perception that was without any genuine 'emotional warmth' for James.

The instantaneous understanding of the emotions of others, rendered possible by the emotional mirror neuron system, is a necessary condition for the empathy which lies at the root of most of our more complex inter-individual relationships. However, sharing someone's emotive state at visceromotor level and feeling empathy for that person are two very different things. For example, if we see that someone is in pain, we are not automatically induced to feel compassion for him. This often occurs, but the two processes are distinct in the sense that the latter implies the former, but not vice versa. Furthermore, compassion depends on many factors other than the recognition of pain; just to name a few: who the other person is, what our relationship with him is, whether or not we are able to imagine ourselves in his position, whether we want to assume responsibility for his emotive state, wishes and expectations, and so on. If it is someone we know and love, the emotive mirroring caused by the sight of their plight may provoke our pity or compassion; if on the other hand the person is an enemy or is doing something that constitutes a threat for us, or if we are declared sadists, then the situation changes radically. In all these cases we understand the other's pain, but we do not necessarily experience empathy.

You will remember that in Wicker's experiment the participants were only told to watch the video; they did not receive other instructions. They were not asked to put themselves (figuratively speaking) in the position of the people they saw on the screen, or imagine what they would have experienced had they been in the demonstrators' place. They did not know why they had to watch the demonstrator smelling the contents of the glass. Therefore the fact that the sight of disgust activated the same areas that were activated by direct experience of the evil-smelling substance, shows that the recognition of the emotive state of the other person was both automatic and immediate. The mirror neuron mechanism functioned due only to the presentation of certain visual stimuli, on which the selectivity of the responses exclusively depended.

Once again the parallel with action understanding is useful to clarify the concept. The reader will recall that the direct nature of this understanding gives rise to a potentially shared space for action, which underlies progressively more elaborate forms of interaction (imitation, intentional communication, etc.) that in turn rest on increasingly articulated and complex mirror neuron systems. Likewise, the brain's capacity to echo the perception of the faces and gestures of others and code them immediately in visceromotor terms, supplies the neural substrate for an empathic sharing that, albeit in different ways and at diverse levels, substantiates and directs our conduct and our inter-individual relationships. Here, too, it is reasonable to expect that the mirror neuron systems will acquire more complex organization and architecture depending on the complexity and sophistication of the related emotional behaviour.

The fact remains that these mechanisms have a common functional matrix similar to that which intervenes in the understanding of actions. Whichever cortical areas are involved, whether motor or visceromotor centres, and what-ever the type of mirroring induced, at neural level the mirror neuron mechanism embodies that modality of understanding which, prior to any form of conceptual and linguistic mediation, gives substance to our experience of others.

Starting from the simple act of picking up a cup of coffee, we have analysed the organization of the motor system and its functionalities, identifying the neural circuits which regulate our interaction with the objects that surround us. The clarification of the nature and reach of the mirror neuron systems then provided us with a base from which to investigate the cerebral processes responsible for the vast range of behaviour that characterizes our daily existence, and from which we weave the web of our social and inter-individual relations.

Bibliography

ADOLPHS, R. (2001), 'The neurobiology of social cognition'. In Current Opinion in Neurobiology, 11, pp. 231–239.

ADOLPHS, R. (2002), 'Neural systems for recognizing emotion'. In Current Opinion in Neurobiology, 12, pp. 169–177.

ADOLPHS, R. (2003), 'Cognitive neuroscience of human social behavior'. In Nature Reviews Neuroscience, 4, pp. 165–178.

ADOLPHS, R., TRANEL, D., DAMASIO, A.R. (2003), 'Dissociable neural systems for recognizing emotions'. In Brain and Cognition, 52, pp. 61–69.

AGLIOTI, S., SMANIA, N., MANFREDI, M., BERLUCCHI, G. (1996), 'Disownership of left hand and objects related to it in a patient with right brain damage'. In Neuroreport, 8, pp. 293–296.

ALLISON, T., PUCE, A., MCCARTHY, G. (2000), 'Social perception from visual cues: role of the STS region'. In Trends in Cognitive Sciences, 4, pp. 267–278.

ALTSCHULER, E.L., VANKOV, A., WANG, V., RAMACHANDRAN, V.S., PINEDA, J.A. (1997), 'Person see, person do: human cortical electrophysiological correlates of monkey see monkey do cell'. In Society of Neuroscience Abstracts, 719.17.

ALTSCHULER, E.L., VANKOV, A., HUBBARD, E.M., ROBERTS, E., RAMACHANDRAN, V.S., PINEDA, J.A. (2000), 'Mu wave blocking by observation of movement and its possible use as a tool to study theory of other minds'. In Society of Neuroscience Abstracts, 68.1.

ANDERSEN, R.A. (1987), 'Inferior parietal lobule function in spatial perception and visuomotor integration'. In BROOKHART, J.M., MOUNTCASTLE, V.B. (editors), Handbook of Physiology. The Nervous System. Higher Function of the Brain. Section 1, vol. 5, American Physiological Society, Bethesda (MD), pp. 483–518.

ANDERSEN, R.A., SNYDER, A.L., BRADLEY, D.C., XING, J. (1997), 'Multimodal representation of space in the posterior parietal cortex and its use in planning movements'. In Annual Review of Neuroscience, 20, pp. 303–330.

ARBIB, M.A. (1981), 'Perceptual structures and distributed motor control'. In BROOKS, V.B. (editor), Handbook of Physiology. Section 2: The Nervous System. Vol.II: Motor Control. Williams and Wilkins, Baltimore, pp. 1449–1480.

ARBIB, M.A. (2002), 'Beyond the mirror system: imitation and evolution of language'. In NEHANIV, C., DAUTENHAHN, K. (editors), Imitation in Animals and Artifacts. MIT Press, Boston (MA), pp. 229–280.

ARBIB, M.A. (2005), 'From monkey-like action recognition to human language: an evolutionary framework for neurolinguistics'. In The Behavioral and Brain Sciences, 28, pp. 105–167.

ARMSTRONG, D.F. (1999), Original Signs. Gesture, Sign and the Sources of Language. Gallauder, Washington.

ARMSTRONG, D.F., STOKOE, W.C., WILCOX, S.E. (1995), Gesture and the Nature of Language. Cambridge University Press, Cambridge.

AUGUSTINE, J.R. (1996), 'Circuitry and functional aspects of the insular lobe in primates including humans'. In Brain Research Reviews, 22, pp. 229–244.

BEKKERING, H. (2002), 'Imitation: common mechanisms in the observation and execution of finger and mouth movements'. In PRINZ, W., MELTZOFF, A.N. (editors), The Imitative Mind: Development, Evolution and Brain Bases. Cambridge University Press, Cambridge, pp. 163–182.

BEKKERING, H., WOHLSCHLÄGER, A. (2002), 'Action perception and imitation: a tutorial'. In PRINZ, W., HOMMEL, B. (editors), Attention and Performance XIX: Common Mechanisms in Perception and Action. Oxford University Press, Oxford, pp. 294–333.

BEKKERING, H., WOHLSCHLÄGER, A., GATTIS, M. (2000), 'Imitation of gestures in children is goal-directed'. In The Quarterly Journal of Experimental Psychology, 53A, pp. 153–164.

BERTHOZ, A. (1997), The Sense of Movement. Editions Odile Jacob, Paris.

BERTI, A., FRASSINETTI, F. (2000), 'When far becomes near: re-mapping of space by tool use'. In Journal of Cognitive Neuroscience, 12, pp. 415–420.

BERTI, A., RIZZOLATTI, G. (1992), 'Visual processing without awareness: evidence from unilateral neglect'. In Journal of Cognitive Neuroscience, 4, pp. 345–351.

BERTI, A., RIZZOLATTI, G. (2002), 'Coding near and far space'. In KARNATH, H.-O., MILNER, D., VALLAR, G. (editors), The Cognitive and Neural Bases of Spatial Neglect. Oxford University Press, Oxford, pp. 119–129.

BERTI, A., SMANIA, N., ALLPORT, A. (2001), 'Coding of far and near space in neglect patients'. In Neuroimage, 14, pp. 98–102.

BICKERTON, D. (1995), Language and Human Behavior. University of Washington Press, Washington.

BINKOFSKI, F., DOHLE, C., POSSE, S., STEPHAN, K.M., HEFTER, H., SEITZ, R.J., FREUND, H.J. (1998), 'Human anterior intraparietal area subserves prehension: a combined lesion and functional MRI activation study'. In Neurology, 50, pp. 1253–1259.

BINKOFSKI, F., BUCCINO, G., POSSE, S., SEITZ, R.J., RIZZOLATTI, G., FREUND, H.J. (1999), 'A fronto-parietal circuit for object manipulation in man: evidence from an fMRI study'. In The European Journal of Neuroscience, 11, pp. 3276–3286.

BISIACH, E., VALLAR, G. (2000), 'Unilateral neglect in humans'. In BOLLER, F., GRAFMAN, J., RIZZOLATTI, G. (editors), Handbook of Neuropsychology, 2a ed. Elsevier, Amsterdam, vol. 1, pp. 459–502.

BLAKEMORE, S.J., DECETY, J. (2001), 'From the perception of action to the understanding of intention'. In Nature Neuroscience, 2, pp. 561–567.

BONIN, VON G., BAILEY, P. (1947), The Neocortex of Macaca Mulatta. University of Illinois Press, Urbana (IL).

BREMMER, F., SCHLACK, A., SHAH, N.J., ZAFIRIS, O., KUBISCHIK, M., HOFFMANN, K., ZILLES, K., FINK, G.R. (2001), 'Polymodal motion processing in posterior parietal and premotor cortex: a human fMRI study strongly implies equivalencies between humans and monkeys'. In Neuron, 29, pp. 287–296.

BRETHERTON, I., FRITZ, J., ZAHN-WAXLER, C., RIDGEWAY, D. (1986), 'The acquisition and development of emotion language: a functionalist perspective'. In Child Development, 57, pp. 529–548.

BRODMANN, K. (1909), Vergleichende Lokalisationslehre der Grosshirnrinde in ihren Prinzipien dargestellt auf Grund des Zellenbaues. Barth, Leipzig.

BRUCE, C.J. (1988), 'Single neuron activity in the monkey's prefrontal cortex'. In RAKIC, P., SINGER, W. (editors), Neurobiology of Neocortex, Wiley, New York, pp. 297–329.

BRUCE, C.J., DESIMONE, R., GROSS, C.G. (1981), 'Visual properties of neurons in a polisensory area in superior temporal sulcus of the macaque'. In Journal of Neurophysiology, 46, pp. 369–384.

BUBNER, R. (1976), Handlung, Sprache und Vernunft. Grundbegriffe praktischer Philosophie, Suhrkamp, Frankfurt am Main.

BUCCINO, G., BINKOFSKI, F., FINK, G.R., FADIGA, L., FOGASSI, L., GALLESE, V., SEITZ, R.J., ZILLES, K., RIZZOLATTI, G., FREUND, H.-J. (2001), 'Action observation activates premotor and parietal areas in a somatotopic manner: an fMRI study'. In The European Journal of Neuroscience, 13, pp. 400–404.

BUCCINO, G., LUI, F., CANESSA, N., PATTERI, I., LAGRAVINESE, G., BENUZZI, F., PORRO, C.A., RIZZOLATTI, G. (2004a), 'Neural circuits involved in the recognition of actions performed by non con-specifics: an fMRI study'. In Journal of Cognitive Neuroscience, 16, pp. 114–126.

BUCCINO, G., VOGT, S., RITZL, A., FINK, G.R., ZILLES, K., FREUND, H.-J., RIZZOLATTI, G. (2004b), 'Neural circuits underlying imitation learning of hand actions: an event-related fMRI study'. In Neuron, 42, pp. 323–334.

BUTTERWORTH, G., HARRIS, M. (1994), Principles of Developmental Psychology. Lawrence Erlbaum Associates, Hove, East Sussex (UK).

BYRNE, R.W. (1995), The Thinking Ape. Evolutionary Origins of Intelligence. Oxford University Press, Oxford.

BYRNE, R.W. (2002), 'Seeing actions as hierarchically organized structures: great ape manual skills'. In PRINZ, W.,

MELTZOFF, A.N. (editors), The Imitative Mind: Development, Evolution and Brain Bases. Cambridge University Press, Cambridge, pp. 122–140.

BYRNE, R.W. (2003), 'Imitation as behaviour parsing'. In Philosophical Transactions of the Royal Society of London, Series B, 358, pp. 529–536.

BYRNE, R.W., RUSSON, A.E. (1998), 'Learning by imitation: a hierarchical approach'. In The Behavioral and Brain Sciences, 21, pp. 667–712.

CALDER, A.J., KEANE, J., MANES, F., ANTOUN, N., YOUNG, A.W. (2000), 'Impaired recognition and experience of disgust following brain injury'. In Nature Neuroscience, 3, pp. 1077–1078.

CALDER, A.J., LAWRENCE, A.D., YOUNG, A.W. (2001), 'Neuropsychology of fear and loathing'. In Nature Reviews Neuroscience, 2, pp. 352–363.

CALVO-MERINO, B., GLASER, D.E., GRÉZES, J., PASSINGHAM, R.E., HAGGARD, P. (2005), 'Action observation and acquired motor skills: an fMRI study with expert dancers'. In Cerebral Cortex, 15, 8, pp. 1243–1249.

CAMINITI, R., FERRAINA, S., JOHNSON, P.B. (1996), 'The sources of visual information to the primate frontal lobe: a novel role for the superior parietal lobule'. In Cerebral Cortex, 6, pp. 319–328.

CAMPBELL, A.W. (1905), Histological Studies on the Localization of Cerebral Function. Cambridge University Press, Cambridge.

CHANGEUX, J.-P., RICOEUR, P. (1998), La nature et la régle: Ce qui fait que nous pensons. Paris, Odile Jacob.

CHAO, L.L., MARTIN, A. (2000), 'Representation of manipulable man-made objects in the dorsal stream'. In Neuroimage, 12, pp. 478–484.

CHENEY, D.L., SEYFARTH, R.M. (1990), How Monkeys See the World. Inside the Mind of Another Species. University of Chicago Press, Chicago/London.

CHIARUGI, G. (1954), Istituzioni di anatomia dell'uomo. Società editrice libraria, Milano.

CHIEFFI, S., FOGASSI, L., GALLESE, V., GENTILUCCI, M. (1992), 'Prehension movements directed to approaching objects: influence of stimulus velocity on the transport and the grasp components'. In Neuropsychologia, 30, pp. 877–897.

COCHIN, S., BARTHELEMY, C., LEJEUNE, B., ROUX, S., MARTINEAU, J. (1998), 'Perception of motion and qEEG activity in human adults'. In Electroencephalography and Clinical Neurophysiology, 107, pp. 287–295.

COCHIN, S., BARTHELEMY, B., ROUX, S., MARTINEAU, J. (1999), 'Observation and execution of movement: similarities demonstrated by quantified electroencephalography'. In The European Journal of Neuroscience, 11, pp. 1839–1842.

COHEN-SEAT, G., GASTAUT, H.J., FAURE, J., HEUYER, G. (1954), 'Études expérimentales de l'activité nerveuse pendant la projection cinématographique'. In Revue International de Filmologie, 5, pp. 7–64.

COLBY, C.L., DUHAMEL, J.-R. (1991), 'Heterogeneity of extrastriate visual areas and multiple parietal areas in the macaque monkeys'. In Neuropsychologia, 29, pp. 517–537.

COLBY, C.L., GOLDBERG, M.E. (1999), 'Space and attention in parietal cortex'. In Annual Review of Neuroscience, 22, pp. 319–349.

COLBY, C.L., GATTASS, R., OLSON, C.R., GROSS, C.G. (1988), 'Topographical organization of cortical afferents to extrastriate visual area PO in the macaque: a dual tracer study'. In The Journal of Comparative Neurology, 269, pp. 392–413.

COLBY, C.L., DUHAMEL, J.-R., GOLDBERG, M.E. (1993), 'Ventral intraparietal area of the macaque: anatomic location and visual response properties'. In Journal of Neurophysiology, 69, pp. 902–914.

CONDILLAC, E. BONNOT DE (1746), An Essay on the Origin of Human Knowledge; being a supplement to Mr. Locke's Essay on the Human Understanding. Engl. Trans. Gainesville, Fla: Scholars' Facsimiles and Reprints 1971.

CORBALLIS, M.C. (1992), 'On the evolution of language and generativity'. In Cognition, 44, pp. 197–226.

CORBALLIS, M.C. (2002), From Hand to Mouth: The Origins of Language. Princeton University Press, Princeton.

CORBALLIS, M.C. (2003), 'From hand to mouth: gestures, speech, and the evolution of right-handedness'. In The Behavioral and Brain Sciences, 26, pp. 199–260.

COWEY, A., SMALL, M., ELLIS, S. (1994), 'Left visual-spatial neglect can be worse in far than in near space'. In Neuropsychologia, 32, pp. 1059–1066.

COWEY, A., SMALL, M., ELLIS, S. (1999), 'No abrupt change in visual hemineglect from near to far space'. In Neuropsychologia, 37, pp. 1–6.

CRAIG, A.D. (2002), 'How do you feel? Interoception: the sense of the physiological condition of the body'. In Nature Reviews of Neuroscience, 4, pp. 2051–2062.

DAMASIO, A.R. (2003), Looking for Spinoza: Joy, Sorrow and the Feeling Brain. Harcourt, New York.

DARWIN, C.R. (1872), The Expression of the Emotions in Man and Animals. John Murray, London. First edition.

DECETY, J., PERANI, D., JEANNEROD, M., BETTINARDI, V., TADARY, B., WOODS, R., MAZZIOTTA, J.C., FAZIO, F. (1994), 'Mapping motor representations with positron emission tomography'. In Nature, 371, pp. 600–602.

DE RENZI, E. (1982), Disorders of Space Exploration and Cognition. John Wiley, Chichester (UK).

DESIMONE, R., ALBRIGHT, T.D., GROSS, C.G., BRUCE, C. (1984), 'Stimulus selective properties of inferior temporal neurons in the macaque'. In Journal of Neuroscience, 4, pp. 2051–2062.

DE WAAL, F.B.M. (1982), Chimpanzee Politics. Power and Sex among Apes. Harper & Row, New York.

DI PELLEGRINO, G., FADIGA, L., FOGASSI, L., GALLESE, V., RIZZOLATTI, G. (1992), 'Understanding motor events: a neurophysiological study'. In Experimental Brain Research, 91, pp. 176–180.

DI PELLEGRINO, G., LÀDAVAS, E., FARNÉ, A. (1997), 'Seeing where your hands are'. In Nature, 388, p. 730.

DONALD, M. (1991), 'Origins of the modern mind: three stages in the evolution of cognition and culture'.

ECONOMO, C. VON, KOSKINAS, G.N. (1925), Die Cytoarchitektonik der Hirnrinde des erwachsenen Menschen. Springer, Wien.

EHRSSON, H.H., FAGERGREN, A., JONSSON, T., WESTLING, G., JOHANSSON, R.S., FORSSBERG, H. (2000), 'Cortical activity in precision- versus power-grip tasks: an fMRI study'. In Journal of Neurophysiology, 83, pp. 528–536.

EVARTS, E.V., SHINODA, Y., WISE, S.P. (1984), Neurophysiological Approaches to Higher Brain Functions. Wiley, New York.

FADIGA, L., FOGASSI, L., PAVESI, G., RIZZOLATTI, G. (1995), 'Motor facilitation during action observation: a magnetic stimulation study'. In Journal of Neurophysiology, 73, pp. 2608–2611.

FADIGA, L., FOGASSI, L., GALLESE, V., RIZZOLATTI, G. (2000), 'Visuomotor neurons: ambiguity of the discharge or 'motor' perception?'. In International Journal of Psychophysiology, 35, pp. 165–177.

FADIGA, L., CRAIGHERO, L., BUCCINO, G., RIZZOLATTI, G. (2002), 'Speech listening specifically modulates the excitability of tongue muscles: a TMS study'. In The European Journal of Neuroscience, 17, pp. 1703–1714.

FAGG, A.H., ARBIB, M.A. (1998), 'Modelling parietal-premotor interactions in primate control grasping'. In Neural Networks, 11, pp. 1277–1308.

FALK, D. (1983), 'The Taung endocast: a reply to Holloway'. In American Journal of Physical Anthropology, 60, pp. 17–45.

FERRARI, P.F., GALLESE, V., RIZZOLATTI, G., FOGASSI, L. (2003), 'Mirror neurons responding to the observation of ingestive and communicative mouth actions in the monkey ventral premotor cortex'. In The European Journal of Neuroscience, 17, pp. 1703–1714.

FIELD, T., WOODSON, R., GREENBERG, R., COHEN, D. (1982), 'Discrimination and imitation of facial expressions by neonates'. In Science, 218, pp. 179–181.

FOGASSI, L., FERRARI, P.F. (2005), 'Neurones miroir, gestes et évolution du langage'. In Primatologie, 6, pp. 263–286.

FOGASSI, L., GALLESE, V. (2002), 'The neural correlates of action understanding in non-human primates'. In STAMENOV, M.I., GALLESE, V. (editors), Mirror Neurons and the Evolution of Brain and Language. Advances in Consciousness Research. John Benjamins Publishing & Co., Amsterdam, pp. 13–55.

FOGASSI, L., GALLESE, V., DI PELLEGRINO, G., FADIGA, L., GENTILUCCI, M., LUPPINO, G., MATELLI, M., PEDOTTI, A., RIZZOLATTI, G. (1992), 'Space coding by premotor cortex'. In Experimental Brain Research, 89, pp. 686–690.

FOGASSI, L., GALLESE, V., FADIGA, L., LUPPINO, G., MATELLI, M., RIZZOLATTI, G. (1996a), 'Coding of peripersonal space in inferior premotor cortex (F4)'. In Journal of Neurophysiology, 76, pp. 141–157.

FOGASSI, L., GALLESE, V., FADIGA, L., RIZZOLATTI, G. (1996b), 'Space coding in inferior premotor cortex (area F4): facts and speculations'. In LACQUANITI, F., VIVIANI, P. (editors), Neural Bases of Motor Behaviour. Kluwer, Dordrecht, pp. 99–120.

FOGASSI, L., GALLESE, V., FADIGA, L., RIZZOLATTI, G. (1998), 'Neurons responding to the sight of goal-directed hand/arm actions in the parietal area PF (7b) of the macaque monkey'. In Society for Neuroscience Abstracts, 24, 257.5.

FOGASSI, L., GALLESE, V., BUCCINO, G., CRAIGHERO, L., FADIGA, L., RIZZOLATTI, G. (2001), 'Cortical mechanisms for the visual guidance of hand grasping movements in the monkey: a reversible inactivation study'. In Brain, 124, pp. 571–586.

FOGASSI, L., FERRARI, P.F., GESIERICH, B., ROZZI, S., CHERSI, F., RIZZOLATTI, G. (2005), 'Parietal lobe: from action organization to intention understanding'. In Science, 308, pp. 662–667.

FRASSINETTI, F., ROSSI, M., LÀDAVAS, E. (2001), 'Passive limb movements improve visual neglect'. In Neuropsychologia, 39, pp. 725–733.

FREUND, H.-J. (1996), 'Historical Overview'. In LUDERS, H.O. (editor), Supplementary Sensorimotor Area. Lippincott-Raven Publishing, Philadelphia, pp. 17–27.

FRONTERA, J.G. (1956), 'Some results obtained by electrical stimulation of the cortex of the island of Reil in the brain of the monkey (Macaca mulatta)'. In The Journal of Comparative Neurology, 105, pp. 365–394.

FUNAHASHI, S., BRUCE, C.J., GOLDMAN-RAKIC, P.S. (1990), 'Mnemonic coding of visual space in the monkey's dorsolateral prefrontal cortex'. In Journal of Neurophysiology, 63, pp. 814–831.

FUSTER, J. M. (1989), The Prefrontal Cortex. Raven Press, New York.

FUSTER, J.M., ALEXANDER, G.E. (1971), 'Neuron activity related to short-term memory'. In Science, 173, pp. 652–654.

GALEA, M.P., DARIAN-SMITH, I. (1994), 'Multiple corticospinal neuron populations in the macaque monkey are specified by their unique cortical origins, spinal terminations, and connections'. In Cerebral Cortex, 4, pp. 166–194.

GALLESE, V. (2000), 'The inner sense of action. Agency and motor representations'. In Journal of Consciousness Studies, 7, 10, pp. 23–40.

GALLESE, V. (2001), 'The "shared manifold" hypothesis: from mirror neuron to empathy'. In Journal of Consciousness Studies, 8, pp. 33–50.

GALLESE, V. (2005), 'Embodied simulation: from neurons to phenomenal experience'. In Phenomenology and the Cognitive Sciences, 4, pp. 23–48.

GALLESE, V., MURATA, A., KASEDA, M., NIKI, N., SAKATA, H. (1994), 'Deficit of hand preshaping after muscimol injection in monkey parietal cortex'. In Neuroreport, 5, pp. 1525–1529.

GALLESE, V., FADIGA, L., FOGASSI, L., RIZZOLATTI, G. (1996), 'Action recognition in the premotor cortex'. In Brain, 119, pp. 593–609.

GALLESE, V., CRAIGHERO, L., FADIGA, L., FOGASSI, L. (1999), 'Perception through action'. In Psyche, 5, p. 21.

GALLESE, V., FOGASSI, L., FADIGA, L., RIZZOLATTI, G. (2002), 'Action representation and the inferior parietal lobule'. In PRINZ, W., HOMMEL, B. (editors), Attention and Performance XIX: Common Mechanisms in Perception and Action. Oxford University Press, Oxford, pp. 335–355.

GALLESE, V., KEYSERS, C., RIZZOLATTI, G. (2004), 'A unifying view of the basis of social cognition'. In Trends in Cognitive Sciences, 8, 9, pp. 396–403.

GALLETTI, C., FATTORI, P., KUTZ, D.F., BATTAGLINI, P.P. (1999), 'Brain location and visual topography of cortical area V6A in the macaque monkey'. In The European Journal of Neuroscience, 11, pp. 575–582.

GALLETTI, C., GAMBERINI, M., KUTZ, D.F., FATTORI, P., LUPPINO, G., MATELLI, M. (2001), 'The cortical connections of area V6A: an occipito-parietal network processing visual information'. In The European Journal of Neuroscience, 13, pp. 1572–1588.

GAMBERINI, M., GALLETTI, C., LUPPINO, G., MATELLI, M. (2002), 'Cytoarchitectonic organization of the functionally defined areas V6 and V6A in the parieto-occipital cortex of macaque brain'. In Journal of Physiology, 543P, 113P.

GANGITANO, M., MOTTAGHY, F.M., PASCUAL-LEONE, A. (2001), 'Phase specific modulation of cortical motor output during movement observation'. In Neuroreport, 12, pp. 1489–1492.

GASTAUT, H.J., BERT, J. (1954), 'EEG changes during cinematographic presentation'. In Electroencephalography and Clinical Neurophysiology, 6, pp. 433–444.

GENTILUCCI, M. (2003), 'Grasp observation influences speech production'. In The European Journal of Neuroscience, 17, pp. 179–184.

GENTILUCCI, M., SCANDOLARA, C., PIGAREV, I.N., RIZZOLATTI, G. (1983), 'Visual responses in the postarcuate cortex (area 6) of the monkey that are independent of eye position'. In Experimental Brain Research, 50, pp. 464–468.

GENTILUCCI, M., FOGASSI, L., LUPPINO, G., MATELLI, M., CAMARDA, R., RIZZOLATTI, G. (1988), 'Functional organization of inferior area 6 in the macaque monkey. I. Somatotopy and the control of proximal movements'. In Experimental Brain Research, 71, pp. 475–490.

GENTILUCCI, M., BENUZZI, F., GANGITANO, M., GRIMALDI, S. (2001), 'Grasp with hand and mouth: a kinematic study on healthy subjects'. In Journal of Neurophysiology, 86, pp. 1685–1699.

GIBSON, J.J. (1979), The Ecological Approach to Visual Perception. Boston, Houghton Mifflin.

GIBSON, K.R., JESSEE, S. (1999), 'Language evolution and expansions of multiple neurological processing areas'. In KING, B.J. (editor), The Origins of Language. What Nonhuman Primates Can Tell Us. School of American Research Press, Santa Fe (NM), pp. 189–227.

GODSCHALK, M., LEMON, R.N., KUYPERS, H.G., RONDAY, H.K (1984), 'Cortical afferents and efferents of monkey postarcuate area: an anatomical and electrophysiological study'. In Experimental Brain Research, 56, pp. 410–424.

GOLDBERG, M.E., BRUCE, C.J. (1990), 'Primate frontal eye fields. III. Maintenance of a spatially accurate saccade signal'. In Journal of Neurophysiology, 64, pp. 489–508.

GOLDBERG, M.E., COLBY, C.L., DUHAMEL, J.-R. (1990), 'The representation of visuomotor space in the parietal lobe of the monkey'. In Cold Spring Harbor Symposia on Quantitative Biology, 55, pp. 729–739.

GOODALE, M.A., MILNER, A.D. (1992), 'Separate visual pathways for perception and action'. In Trends in Neurosciences, 15 pp. 20–25.

GOODALL, J. (1986), The Chimpanzees of Gombe: Patterns of Behavior. Harvard University Press, Cambridge (MA).

GRAFTON, S.T., ARBIB, M.A., FADIGA, L., RIZZOLATTI, G. (1996), 'Localization of grasp representations in humans by PET: 2. Observation compared with imagination'. In Experimental Brain Research, 112, pp. 103–111.

GRAFTON, S.T., FADIGA, L., ARBIB, M.A., RIZZOLATTI, G. (1997), 'Premotor cortex activation during observation and naming of familiar tools'. In Neuroimage, 6, pp. 231–236.

GRAZIANO, M.S.A., GROSS, C.G. (1994), 'Mapping space with neurons'. In Current Directions in Psychological Science, 3, 5, pp.164–167.

GRAZIANO, M.S.A., GROSS, C.G. (1995), 'The representation of extrapersonal space. A possible role for bimodal, visual-tactile neurons'. In GAZZANIGA, M.S. (editor), The Cognitive Neurosciences. MIT Press, Cambridge (MA).

GRAZIANO, M.S.A., GROSS, C.G. (1998), 'Spatial maps for the control of movement'. In Current Opinion in Neurobiology, 8, pp. 195–201.

GRAZIANO, M.S.A., YAP, G.S., GROSS, C.G. (1994), 'Coding of visual space by premotor neurons'. In Science, 266, pp. 1054–1057.

GRAZIANO, M.S.A., HU, X., GROSS, C.G. (1997), 'Visuo-spatial properties of ventral premotor cortex'. In Journal of Neurophysiology, 77, pp. 2268–2292.

GRAZIANO, M.S.A., REISS, L.A.J., GROSS, C.G. (1999), 'A neural representation of the location of nearby sounds'. In Nature, 397, pp. 428–430.

GREENWALD, A.G. (1970), 'Sensory feedback mechanisms in performance control: with special reference to the ideomotor mechanism'. In Psychological Review, 77, pp. 73–99.

GRÉZES, J., DECETY, J. (2001), 'Functional anatomy of execution, mental simulation, observation and verb generation of actions: a meta-analysis'. In Human Brain Mapping, 12, pp. 1–19.

GRÉZES, J., COSTES, N., DECETY, J. (1998), 'Top-down effect of strategy on the perception of human biological motion: a PET investigation'. In Cognitive Neuropsychology, 15, pp. 553–582.

HADAR, U., WENKERT-OLENIK, D., KRAUSS, R., SOROKER, N. (1998), 'Gesture and processing of the speech: neuropsychological evidence'. In Brain and Language, 62, pp. 107–126.

HALLIGAN, P.W., MARSHALL, J.C. (1991), 'Left neglect for near but not far space in man'. In Nature, 350, pp. 498–500.

HANLON, R.E., BROWN, J.W., GERSTMAN, L.J. (1990), 'Enhancement of naming in nonfluent aphasia through gesture'. In Brain and Language, 38, pp. 298–314.

HARI, R., FORSS, N., AVIKAINEN, S., KIRVESKARI, S., SALENIUS, S., RIZZOLATTI, G. (1998), 'Activation of human primary motor cortex during action observation: a neuromagnetic study'. In Proceedings of National Academy of Sciences of the United States of America, 95, pp. 15061–15065.

HAUSER, M.D. (1996), The Evolution of Communication. MIT Press, Cambridge (MA).

HAUSER, M.D., CHOMSKY, N., FITCH, W.T. (2002), 'The faculty of language: what is it, who has it, and how did it evolve?'. In Science, 286, pp. 2526–2528.

HE, S.Q., DUM, R.P., STRICK, P.L. (1993), 'Topographic organization of corticospinal projections from the frontal lobe: motor areas on the lateral surface of the hemisphere'. In Journal of Neuroscience, 13, pp. 952–980.

HE, S.Q., DUM, R.P., STRICK, P.L. (1995), Topographic organization of corticospinal projections from the frontal lobe: motor areas on the medial surface of the hemisphere'. In Journal of Neuroscience, 15, pp. 3284–3306.

HEISER, M., IACOBONI, M., MAEDA, F., MARCUS, J., MAZZIOTTA, J.C.(2003), 'The essential role of Broca's area in imitation'. In The European Journal of Neuroscience, 17, pp. 1123–1128.

HENNEMAN, E. (1984), 'Organization of the motor system. A preview'. In MOUNTCASTLE, V.B., Medical Physiology, XIV Edition, The C.V. Mosby Company, Saint Louis, pp. 669–673.

HEYES, C. (2001), 'Causes and consequences of imitation'. In Trends in Cognitive Sciences, 5, pp. 253–261.

HOLLOWAY, R.L. (1983), 'Human paleontological evidence relevant to language behavior'. In Human Neurobiology, 2, pp. 105–114.

HOLLOWAY, R.L. (1985), 'The past, present, and future significance of the lunate sulcus in early hominid evolution'. In TOBIAS, P.V. (editor), Hominid Evolution. Past, Present, and Future. Allen R. Liss, New York, pp. 47–62.

HUTCHISON, W.D., DAVIS, K.D., LOZANO, A.M., TASKER, R.R., DOSTROVSKY, J.O. (1999), 'Pain related neurons in the human cingulate cortex'. In Nature Neuroscience, 2, pp. 403–405.

HYVÄRINEN, J. (1981), 'Regional distribution of functions in parietal association area 7 of the monkey'. In Brain Research, 206, pp. 287–303.

IACOBONI, M., WOODS, R.P., BRASS, M., BEKKERING, H., MAZZIOTTA, J.C., RIZZOLATTI, G. (1999), 'Cortical mechanisms of human imitation'. In Science, pp. 2526–2528.

IACOBONI, M., KOSKI, L.M., BRASS, M., BEKKERING, H., WOODS, R.P., DUBEAU, M.C., MAZZIOTTA, J.C., RIZZOLATTI, G. (2001), 'Reafferent copies of imitated actions in the right superior temporal cortex'. In Proceedings of National Academy of Sciences of the United States of America, 98, 24, pp. 13995–13999.

IACOBONI, M., MOLNAR-SZAKACS, I., GALLESE, V., BUCCINO, G., MAZZIOTTA, J.C., RIZZOLATTI, G. (2005), 'Grasping the intentions of others with one's own mirror neuron system'. In PLoS Biology, 3, pp. 529–535.

INGLE, D. (1967), 'Two visual mechanisms underlying the behavior of fish'. In Psychologische Forschung, 31, pp. 44–51.

INGLE, D. (1973), 'Two visual systems in the frog'. In Science, 181, pp. 1053–1055.

IRIKI, A., TANAKA, M., IWAMURA, Y. (1996), 'Coding of modified body schema during tool use by macaque post-central neurons'. In Neuroreport, 7, pp. 2325–2330.

JACOB, P., JEANNEROD, M. (2003), Ways of Seeing. The Scope and Limits of Visual Cognition. Oxford University Press, New York.

JAMES, W. (1890), Principles of Psychology. Holt, Rinehart & Winston, New York.

JEANNEROD, M. (1988), The Neural and Behavioural Organization of Goal-directed Movements. Oxford University Press, Oxford.

JEANNEROD, M. (1994), 'The representing brain: neural correlates of motor intention and imagery'. In Behavioral Brain Sciences, 17, pp. 187–245.

JEANNEROD, M. (1997), The Cognitive Neuroscience of Action. Blackwell, Oxford.

JEANNEROD, M., (2006) Motor Cognition. Oxford University Press. Oxford.

JEANNEROD, M., ARBIB, M.A., RIZZOLATTI, G., SAKATA, H. (1995), 'Grasping objects: the cortical mechanisms of visuomotor transformation'. In Trends in Neuroscience, 18, pp. 314–320.

JELLEMA, T., BAKER, C.I., WICKER, B., PERRETT, D.I. (2000), 'Neural representation for the perception of the intentionality of actions'. In Brain and Cognition, 44, pp. 280–302.

JELLEMA, T., BAKER, C.I., ORAM, M.W., PERRETT, D.I. (2002), 'Cell populations in the banks of the superior temporal sulcus of the macaque monkey and imitation'. In MELTZOFF, A.N., PRINZ, W. (editors), The Imitative Mind: Development, Evolution and Brain Bases. Cambridge University Press, Cambridge, pp. 267–290.

JÜRGENS, U. (1995), 'Neuronal control of vocal production in humans and non humans primates'.

In ZIMMERMAN, E., NEWMAN, J.D., JÜRGENS, U. (editors), Current Topics in Primate Vocal Communication. Plenum Press, New York, pp. 199–206.

JÜRGENS, U. (2002), 'Neural pathways underlying vocal control'. In Neuroscience and Biobehavioral Review, 26, pp. 235–258.

KAADA, B.R., PRIBRAM, K.H., EPSTEIN, J. (1949), 'Respiratory and vascular responses in monkeys from temporal pole, insula, orbital surface and cingulated gyrus'. In Journal of Neurophysiology, 12, pp. 347–356.

KAWATO, M. (1997), 'Bidirectional theory approach to consciousness'. In ITO, M., MIYASHITA, Y., ROLLS, E.T. (editors), Cognition, Computation and consciousness. Oxford University Press, Oxford, pp. 223–248.

KAWATO, M. (1999), 'Internal models for motor control and trajectory planning'. In Current Opinion in Neurobiology, 9, pp. 718–727.

KEIZER, K., KUYPERS, H.G.J.M. (1989), 'Distribution of corticospinal neurons with collaterals to the lower brain stem reticular formation in monkey (Macaca fascicularis)'. In Experimental Brain Research, 74, pp. 311–318.

KEYSERS, C., KOHLER, E., UMILTÀ, M.A., FOGASSI, L., RIZZOLATTI, G., GALLESE, V. (2003), 'Audio-visual mirror neurons and action recognition'. In Experimental Brain Research, 153, pp. 628–636.

KOHLER, E., KEYSERS, C., UMILTÀ, M.A., FOGASSI, L., GALLESE, V., RIZZOLATTI, G. (2002), 'Hearing sounds, understanding actions: action representation in mirror neurons'. In Science, 297, pp. 846–848.

KOSKI, L., WOHLSCHLÄGER, A., BEKKERING, H., WOODS, R.P., DUBEAU, M.C. (2002), 'Modulation of motor and premotor activity during imitation of target-directed actions'. In Cerebral Cortex, 12, pp. 847–855.

KOSKI, L., IACOBONI, M., DUBEAU, M.C., WOODS, R.P., MAZZIOTTA, J.C. (2003), 'Modulation of cortical activity during different imitative behaviors'. In Journal of Neurophysiology, 89, pp. 460–471.

KRAMS, M., RUSHWORTH, M.F., DEIBER, M.P., FRACKOWIAK, R.S., PASSINGHAM, R.E. (1998), 'The preparation, execution and suppression of copied movements in the human brain'. In Experimental Brain Research, 120, pp. 386–398.

KROLAK-SALMON, P., HENAFF, M.A., ISNARD, J., TALLON-BAUDRY, C., GUENOT, M., VIGHETTO, A., BERTRAND, O., MAUGUIERE, F. (2003), 'An attention modulated response to disgust in human ventral anterior insula'. In Annals of Neurology, 53, pp. 446–453.

LACQUANITI, F., GUIGON, E., BIANCHI, L., FERRAINA, S., CAMINITI, R. (1995), 'Representing spatial information for limb movement: role of area 5 in the monkey'. In Cerebral Cortex, 5, pp. 391–409.

LÀDAVAS, E., DI PELLEGRINO, G., FARNÉ, A., ZELONI, G. (1998a), 'Neuropsychological evidence of an integrated visuotactile representation of peripersonal space in humans'. In Journal of Cognitive Neuroscience, 10, pp. 581–589.

LÀDAVAS, E., ZELONI, G., FARNÉ, A. (1998b), 'Visual peripersonal space centred on the face in humans'. In Brain, 121, pp. 2317–2326.

LEINONEN, L., NYMAN, G. (1979), 'II. Functional properties of cells in anterolateral part of area 7 associative face area of awake monkeys'. In Experimental Brain Research, 34, pp. 321–333.

LEINONEN, L., HIVÄRINEN, J., NYMAN, G., LINNANKOSKI, I. (1979), 'I. Function properties of neurons in lateral part of associative area 7 in awake monkeys'. In Experimental Brain Research, 34, pp. 299–320.

LIBERMAN, A.M. (1993), 'Some assumptions about speech and how they changed'. In Haskins Laboratories Status Report on Speech Research, 113, pp. 1–32.

LIEBERMAN, P. (1975), On the Origins of Language. An Introduction to the Evolution of Human Speech. MacMillan Publishing Co., New York.

LIBERMAN, A.M., WHALEN, D.H. (2000), 'On the relation of speech to language'. In Trends in Cognitive Neuroscience, 4, pp. 187–196.

LIVET, P. (1997), 'Modéles de la motricité et théorie de l'action'. In PETIT, J.-L. (editor), Les neurosciences et la philosophie de l'action. Vrin, Paris, pp. 341–361.

LOTZE, H. (1852), Medicinische Psychologie oder Physiologie der Seele. Weidmannsche Buchandlung, Leipzig.

LUPPINO, G., RIZZOLATTI, G. (2000), 'The organization of the frontal motor cortex'. In News in Physiological Sciences, 15, pp. 219–224.

LUPPINO, G., MATELLI, M., CAMARDA, R., GALLESE, V., RIZZOLATTI, G. (1991), 'Multiple representations of body movements in mesial area 6 and the adjacent cingulated cortex: an intercortical microstimulation study'. In The Journal of Comparative Neurology, 311, pp. 463–482.

LUPPINO, G., MATELLI, M., CAMARDA, R., RIZZO-LATTI, G. (1993), 'Corticocortical connections of area F3 (SMA-Proper) and area F6 (Pre-SMA) in the macaque monkey'. In The Journal of Comparative Neurology, 338, pp. 114–140.

LUPPINO, G., MURATA, A., GOVONI, P., MATELLI, M. (1999), 'Largely segregated parietofrontal connections linking rostral intraparietal cortex (areas AIP and VIP) and the ventral premotor cortex (areas F5 and F4)'. In Experimental Brain Research, 128, pp. 181–187.

LURIJA, A.R. (1973), The Working Brain. An Introduction to Neuropsychology. Penguin Books, Harmondsworth.

MACH, E. (1905), Knowledge and Error. Sketches on the Psychology of Enquiry. Engl. Trans. Reidel, Dordrecht 1967.

MACNEILAGE, P.F. (1998), 'The frame/content theory of evolution of speech production'. In The Behavioral and Brain Sciences, 21, pp. 499–511.

MAEDA, F., KLEINER-FISMAN, G., PASCUAL-LEONE, A. (2002), 'Motor facilitation while observing hand actions: specificity of the effect and role of observer's orientation'. In Journal of Neurophysiology, 87, pp. 1329–1335.

MAESTRIPIERI, D. (1996), 'Gestural communication and its cognitive implications in pigtail macaques (Macaca nemestrina)'. In Behaviour, 133, pp. 997–1022.

MARSHALL, J.F., HALLIGAN, P.W. (1988), 'Blindsight and insight in visuo-spatial neglect'. In Nature, 311, pp. 445–462.

MARTIN, A. WIGGS, C.L., UNGERLEIDER, L.G. HAXBY, J.V (1996), 'Neural correlates of category-specific knowledge'. In Nature, 379, pp. 649–652.

MASSARO, D.W. (1990), 'An information-processing analysis of perception and action'. In NEUMANN, O., PRINZ,W. (editors), Relationship between Perception and Action: Current Approaches. Springer, Berlin, pp. 133–166.

MATELLI, M., LUPPINO, G. (1998), 'Functional anatomy of human motor cortical areas'. In BOLLER, F., GRAFMAN, J. (editors), Handbook of Neurophysiology. Elsevier Science, Amsterdam, vol. 11, pp. 9–26.

MATELLI, M., LUPPINO, G., RIZZOLATTI, G. (1985), 'Patterns of cytochrome oxidase activity in the frontal agranular cortex of the macaque monkey'. InBehavioural Brain Research, 18, pp. 125–136.

MATELLI, M., CAMARDA, R., GLICKSTEIN, M., RIZZOLATTI, G. (1986), 'Afferent and efferent projections of the inferior area 6 in the macaque monkey'. In The Journal of Comparative Neurology, 251, pp. 291–298.

MATELLI, M., LUPPINO, G., RIZZOLATTI, G. (1991), 'Architecture of superior and mesial area 6 and of the adjacent cingulate cortex'. In The Journal of Comparative Neurology, 311, pp. 445–462.

MATSUMARA, M., KUBOTA, K. (1979), 'Cortical projection of hand-arm motor area from postarcuate area in macaque monkey: a histological study of retrograde transport of horseradish peroxidase'. In Neuroscience Letters, 11, pp. 241–246.

MEAD, G.H. (1907), 'Concerning animal perception'. In Psychological Review, 14, pp. 383–390.

MEAD, G.H. (1910), 'Social consciousness and the consciousness of meaning'. Psychological Bulletin, 7(12), 398, now also in Selected Writings: George Herbert Mead (1964) edited by Andrew J. Reck, p. 124.

MEAD, G.H. (1938), The Philosophy of the Act. Edited by C.W. Morris, J.M. Brewster, A.M. Dunham, D. Miller, University of Chicago, Chicago (IL).

MEISTER, I.G., BOROOJERDI, B., FOLTYS, H., SPARING, R., HUBER, W., TOPPER, R. (2003), 'Motor cortex hand area and speech: implications for the development of language'. In Neurophysiologia, 41, pp. 401–406.

MELTZOFF, A.N. (2002), 'Elements of a developmental theory of imitation'. In PRINZ, W., MELTZOFF, A.N. (editors), The Imitative Mind: Development, Evolution and Brain Bases. Cambridge University Press, Cambridge, pp. 19–41.

MELTZOFF, A.N., MOORE, M.K. (1977), 'Imitation of facial and manual gestures by human neonates'. In Science, 198, pp. 75–78.

MELTZOFF, A.N., MOORE, M.K. (1997), 'Explaining facial imitation: a theoretical model'. In Early Development and Parenting, 6, pp. 179–192.

MERLEAU-PONTY, M. (1945), Phenomenology of Perception. Engl. Trans. Routledge, London and New York. 2002.

MESULAM, M.M., MUFSON, E.J. (1982a), 'Insula of the old world monkey. I. Architectonics in the insulo-orbito-temporal component of the paralimbic brain'. In The Journal of Comparative Neurology, 212, pp. 1–22.

MESULAM, M.M., MUFSON, E.J. (1982b), 'Insula of the old world monkey. III. Efferent cortical output and comments on function'. In The Journal of Comparative Neurology, 212, pp. 38–52.

MILNER, A.D. (1987), 'Animal model for the syndrome of spatial neglect'. In JEANNEROD, M. (editor), Neurophysiological and Neuropsychological Aspects of Spatial Neglect. North-Holland, Amsterdam, pp. 295–288.

MILNER, A.D., GOODALE, M.A. (1995), The Visual Brain in Action. Oxford University Press, Oxford.

MOUNTCASTLE, V.B. (1995), 'The parietal system and some higher brain functions'. In Cerebral Cortex, 5, pp. 377–390.

MOUNTCASTLE, V.B., LYNCH, J.C, GEORGOPULOS, A., SAKATA, H., ACUNA, C. (1975), 'Posterior parietal association cortex of the monkey: command functions for operations within extrapersonal space'. In Journal of Neurophysiology, 38, pp. 871–908.

MUAKKASSA, K.F., STRICK, P.L. (1979), 'Frontal lobe inputs to primate motor cortex: evidence for four somatotopically organized 'premotor' areas'. In Brain Research, 177, pp. 176–182.

MUFSON, E.J., MESULAM, M.M. (1982), 'Insula of the old world monkey. II. Afferent cortical output and comments on the claustrum'. In The Journal of Comparative Neurology, 212, pp. 23–37.

MURATA, A., GALLESE, V., KASEDA, M., SAKATA, H. (1996), 'Parietal neurons related to memory-guided hand manipulation'. In Journal of Neurophysiology, 75, pp. 2180–2185.

MURATA, A., FADIGA, L., FOGASSI, L., GALLESE, V., RAOS, V., RIZZOLATTI, G. (1997), 'Object representation in the ventral premotor cortex (area F 5) of the monkey'. In Journal of Neurophysiology, 78, pp. 2226–2230.

MURATA, A., GALLESE, V., LUPPINO, G., KASEDA, M., SAKATA, H. (2000), 'Selectivity for the shape, size and orientation of objects for grasping in neurons of monkey parietal area AIP'. In Journal of Neurophysiology, 79, pp. 2580–2601.

NELISSEN, K., LUPPINO G., VANDUFFEL,W., RIZZOLATTI, G., ORBAN, G.A. (2005), 'Observing others: multiple action representation in the frontal lobe'. In Science, 14, 310, pp. 332–336.

NISHITANI, N., HARI, R. (2000), 'Temporal dynamics of cortical representation for action'. In Proceedings of National Academy of Sciences of the United States of America, 97, pp. 913–918.

NISHITANI, N., HARI, R. (2002), 'Viewing lip forms: cortical dynamics'. In Neuron, 36, pp. 1211–1220.

PAGET, R. (1930), Human Speech. Keegan Paul, London.

PANDYA, D.N., SELTZER, B. (1982), 'Intrinsic connection-sand architectonics of posterior parietal cortex in rhesus monkey'. In The Journal of Comparative Neurology, 204, pp. 196–210.

PASSINGHAM, R.E. (1993), The Frontal Lobe and Voluntary Action. Oxford University Press, Oxford.

PASSINGHAM, R.E., TONI, I., RUSHWORTH, M.F.S. (2000), 'Specialisation within the prefrontal cortex: the ventral prefrontal cortex and associative learning'. In Experimental Brain Research, 133, pp. 103–113.

PENFIELD, W., FAULK, M.E. (1955), 'The insula: further observations on its function'. In Brain, 78, pp. 445–470.

PENFIELD, W., RASMUSSEN, T. (1950), The Cerebral Cortex of Man. A Clinical Study of Localization of Function, Macmillan, New York.

PERANI, D., CAPPA, S.F., BETTINARDI, V. (1995), 'Different neural systems for the recognition of animals and man-made tools'. In Neuroreport, 6, pp. 1637–1641.

PERRETT, D.I., ROLLS, E.T., CAAN, W. (1982), 'Visual neurons responsive to faces in the monkey temporal cortex'. In Experimental Brain Research, 47, pp. 329–342.

PERRETT, D.I., SMITH, P.A.J., POTTER, D.D., MISTLING, A.J., HEAD, A.S., MILNER, A.D., JEVES, M.A. (1984), 'Neurons responsive to faces in the temporal cortex: studies of functional organization, sensitivity to identity and relation to perception'. In Human Neurobiology, 3, pp. 197–208.

PERRETT, D.I., SMITH, P.A.J., POTTER, D.D., MISTLING, A.J., HEAD, A.S., MILNER, A.D., JEVES, M.A. (1985), 'Visual cells in the temporal cortex sensitive to face view and gaze direction'. In Proceedings of Royal

Society of London Series B Biological Sciences, 223, pp. 293–317.

PERRETT, D.I., HARRIES, M.H., BEVAN, R., THOMAS, S., BENSON, P.J., MISTLIN, A.J., CHITTY, A.J., HIETANEN, J.K., ORTEGA, J.E. (1989), 'Frameworks of analysis for the neural representation of animate objects and actions'. In Journal of Experimental Biology, 146, pp. 87–113.

PERRETT, D.I., MISTLIN, A.J., HARRIES, M.H., CHITTY, A.J. (1990), 'Understanding the visual appearance and consequence of hand actions'. In GOODALE, M.A. (editor), Vision and Action: The Control of Grasping. Ablex, Norwood, pp. 163–180.

PETIT, J.-L. (1999), 'Constitution by movement: Husserl in light of recent neurobiological findings'. In PETITOT, J., VARELA, F.J., PACHOUD, B., ROY, J.-M. (editors), Naturalizing Phenomenology: Issues in Contemporary Phenomenology and Cognitive Science. Stanford University Press, Stanford (CA), pp. 220–244.

PETRIDES, M., PANDYA, D.N. (1984), 'Projections to the frontal cortex from the posterior parietal region in the rhesus monkey'. In The Journal of Comparative Neurology, 228, pp. 105–116.

PETRIDES, M., PANDYA, D.N. (1997), 'Comparative architectonic analysis of the human and the macaque frontal cortex'. In BOLLER, F., GRAFMAN, J. (editors), Handbook of Neuropsychology. Elsevier, Amsterdam, vol. 9, pp. 17–58.

PHILLIPS, M.L., YOUNG, A.W., SENIOR, C., BRAMMER, M., ANDREW, C., CALDER, A.J., BULLMORE, E.T., PERRETT, D.I., ROWLAND, D., WILLIAM, S.C., et al. (1997), 'A specific neural substrate for perceiving facial expressions of disgust'. In Nature, 389, pp. 495–498.

PHILLIPS, M.L., YOUNG, A.W., SCOTT, S.K., CALDER, A.J., ANDREW, C., GIAMPIETRO, V., WILLIAM, S.C., BULLMORE, E.T., BRAMMER, M., GRAY, J.A. (1998), 'Neural responses to facial and vocal expressions of fear and disgust'. In Proceedings of Royal Society of London Series B Biological Sciences, 265, pp. 1089–1817.

PIAGET, J. (1936), La naissance de l'intelligenze chez l'enfant. Delachaux et Niestlé, Neuchâtel.

PINKER, S. (1994), The Language Instinct. William Morrow & Company, New York.

POINCARÉ, J.-H. (1908), Science and Method. Engl. Trans. Routledge, London 1996.

POINCARÉ, J.-H. (1913), Derniéres pensées, Edition Ernest Flammarion, Paris.

PORTER, R., LEMON, R. (1993), Corticospinal Function and Voluntary Movement. Clarendon Press, Oxford.

PRINZ, W. (1987), 'Ideomotor action'. In HEUER, H., SANDERS, A.F. (editors), Perspectives on Perception and Action. Erlbaum, Hillsdale (NJ), pp. 47–76.

PRINZ, W. (1990), 'A common-coding approach to perception and action'. In NEUMANN, O., PRINZ, W. (editors), Relationship between Perception and Action: Current Approaches. Springer, Berlin, pp. 167–203.

PRINZ, W. (2002), 'Experimental approaches to imitation'. In PRINZ, W., MELTZOFF, A.N. (editor), The Imitative Mind: Development, Evolution and Brain Bases. Cambridge University Press, Cambridge, pp. 143–162.

RIZZOLATTI, G. (2005), 'The mirror neuron system and imitation'. In HURLEY, S., CHATER, N. (editors), Perspectives on Imitation. From Neuroscience to Social Science. MIT Press, Cambridge (MA), vol. 1, pp. 55–76.

RIZZOLATTI, G., ARBIB, M.A. (1998), 'Language within our grasp'. In Trends in Neuroscience, 21, pp. 188–194.

RIZZOLATTI, G., BERTI A. (1990), 'Neglect as a neural representational deficit'. Revue Neurologique, 146 (10), 624–634.

RIZZOLATTI, G., BERTI, A.. (1993) 'Neural mechanisms of spatial neglect'. In ROBERTSON, I.H., MARSHALL, J.C. (editors), Unilateral Neglect: Clinical and Experimental Studies, 87 105, Taylor & Francis, London(UK).

RIZZOLATTI, G., BUCCINO, G. (2005), 'The mirror neuron system and its role in imitation and language'. In DEHAENE, S., DUHAMEL, J.-R., HAUSER, M.D., RIZZOLATTI, G. (editor), From Monkey Brain to Human Brain. A Fyssen Foundation Symposium. MIT Press, Cambridge (MA), pp. 213–233.

RIZZOLATTI, G., CRAIGHERO, L. (2004), 'The mirror neuron system'. In Annual Reviews of Neuroscience, 27, pp. 169–192.

RIZZOLATTI, G., FADIGA, L. (1998), 'Grasping objects and grasping action meanings: the dual role of monkey rostroventral premotor cortex (area F5)'. In BOCK, G.R., CODE, J.A. (editors), Sensory Guidance of Movement. Novartis Foundation Symposium 218, John Wiley & Sons, Chichester (UK), pp. 269–284.

RIZZOLATTI, G., GALLESE, V. (1988), 'Mechanisms and theories of spatial neglect'. In BOLLETT, F., GRAFMAN, J. (editors), Handbook of Neuropsychology. Elsevier, Amsterdam, vol. 1, pp. 223–246.

RIZZOLATTI, G., GALLESE, V. (1997), 'From action to meaning: a neurophysiological perspective'. In PETIT, J.-L. (editor), Les neurosciences et la philosophie de l'action. Vrin, Paris, pp. 217–229.

RIZZOLATTI, G., GENTILUCCI, M. (1988), 'Motor and visual-motor functions of the premotor cortex'. In RAKIC, P., SINGER, W. (editors), Neurobiology of Neocortex. John Wiley & Sons, Chichester (UK), pp. 269–284.

RIZZOLATTI, G., LUPPINO, G. (2001), 'The cortical motor system'. In Neuron, 31, pp. 889–901.

RIZZOLATTI, G., MATELLI, M. (2003), 'Two different streams form the dorsal visual stream: anatomy and functions'. In Experimental Brain Research, 153, pp. 146–157.

RIZZOLATTI, G., SCANDOLARA, C., GENTILUCCI, M., MATELLI, M. (1981a), 'Afferent properties of periarcuate neurons in macaque monkeys. I. Somatosensory responses'. In Experimental Brain Research, 2, pp. 125–146.

RIZZOLATTI, G., SCANDOLARA, C., MATELLI, M., GENTILUCCI, M. (1981b), 'Afferent properties of periarcuate neurons in macaque monkeys. II. Visual responses'. In Experimental Brain Research, 2, pp. 147–163.

RIZZOLATTI, G., MATELLI, M., PAVESI, G. (1983), 'Deficits in attention and movement following the removal of postarcuate (area 6) and periarcuate (area 8) cortex in macaque monkeys'. In Brain, 206, pp. 655–673.

RIZZOLATTI, G., GENTILUCCI, M., FOGASSI, L., LUPPINO, G., MATELLI, M., PONZONI MAGGI S. (1987), 'Neurons related to goal-directed motor acts in inferior area 6 of the macaque monkey'. In Experimental Brain Research, 67, pp. 220–224.

RIZZOLATTI, G., CAMARDA, R., FOGASSI, L., GENTILUCCI, M., LUPPINO, G., MATELLI, M. (1988), 'Functional organization of area 6 in the macaque monkey. II. Area F5 and the control of distal movements'. In Experimental Brain Research, 71, pp. 491–507.

RIZZOLATTI, G., RIGGIO, L., SHELIGA, B.M. (1994), 'Space and selective attention'. In UMILTÀ, C., MOSCHOVITCH, M. (editor), Attention and Performance XV. MIT Press, Cambridge (MA), pp. 231–265.

RIZZOLATTI, G., FADIGA, L., GALLESE, V., FOGASSI, L. (1996a), 'Premotor cortex and the recognition of motor actions'. In Cognitive Brain Research, 3, pp. 131–141.

RIZZOLATTI, G., FOGASSI, L., MATELLI, M., BETTINARDI, V., PAULESU, E., PERANI, D., FAZIO, F. (1996b), 'Localization of grasp representations in humans by PET: 1. Observation versus execution'. In Experimental Brain Research, 111, pp. 246–252.

RIZZOLATTI, G., FADIGA, L., FOGASSI, L., GALLESE, V. (1997), 'The space around us'. In Science, 277, pp. 190–191.

RIZZOLATTI, G., LUPPINO, G., MATELLI, M. (1998), 'The organization of the cortical motor system: new concepts'. In Electroencephalography and Clinical Neurophysiology, 106, pp. 283–296.

RIZZOLATTI, G., FOGASSI, L., GALLESE, V. (1999a), 'Cortical mechanisms subserving object grasping and action recognition: a new view on the cortical motor functions'. In GAZZANIGA, M.S. (editor), The Cognitive Neurosciences. 2a ed. MIT Press, Cambridge (MA), pp. 539–552.

RIZZOLATTI, G., FADIGA, L., FOGASSI, L., GALLESE, V. (1999b), 'Resonance behaviors and mirror neurons'. In Archives Italiennes de Biologie, 137, pp. 83–99.

RIZZOLATTI, G., BERTI, A., GALLESE, V., (2000) 'Spatial neglect: neurophysiological bases, cortical circuits and theories'. In BOLLER, F., GRAFMAN, J. (editors), Handbook of Neurophysiology. 2a ed., Elsevier, Amsterdam, pp. 503–537.

RIZZOLATTI, G., FOGASSI, L., GALLESE, V. (2001), 'Neurophysiological mechanisms underlying the under-standing and imitation of action'. In Nature Reviews Neuroscience, 2, pp. 661–670.

RIZZOLATTI, G., FOGASSI, L., GALLESE, V. (2002a), 'Motor and cognitive functions of the ventral premotor cortex'. In Current Opinion in Neurobiology, 12, pp. 149–154.

RIZZOLATTI, G., FADIGA, L., FOGASSI, L., GALLESE, V. (2002b), 'From mirror neurons to imitation: facts and speculations'. In MELTZOFF, A.N., PRINZ,W. (editors), The Imitative Mind. Development, Evolution, and Brain Bases. Cambridge University Press, Cambridge, pp. 247–266.

ROWE, J.B., TONI, I., JOSEPHS, O., FRACKOWIACK, R.S., PASSINGHAM, R.E. (2000), 'The prefrontal cortex: response selection or maintenance within working memory'. In Science, 288, pp. 1656–1660.

ROYET, J.P., ZALD, D., VERSACE, R., COSTES, N., LAVENNE, F., KOENIG, O., GERVAIS, R. (2000), 'Emotional responses to pleasant and unpleasant olfac-tory, visual and auditory stimuli: a positron emission tomography study'. In Journal of Neuroscience, 20, pp. 7752–7759.

ROYET, J.P., HUDRY, J., ZALD, D.H., GODINOT, D., GREGOIRE, M.C., LAVENNE, F., COSTES, N., HOLLEY, A. (2001), 'Functional neuroanatomy of differ-ent olfactory judgements'. In Neuroimage, 13, pp. 506–519.

ROYET, J.P., PLAILLY, J., DELON-MARTIN, C., KAREKEN, D.A., SEGEBARTH, C. (2003), 'fMRI of emotional responses to odors: influence of hedonic valence and judgement, handedness, and gender'. In Neuroimage, 20, pp. 713–728.

ROZIN, R., HAIDT, J., MCCAULEY, C.R. (2000), 'Disgust'. In LEWIS, M., HAVILAND-JONES, J.M. (editor), Handbook of Emotions. 2a ed., Guilford Press, New York, pp. 637–653.

SAKATA, H., TAIRA, M., MURATA, A., MINE, S. (1995), 'Neural mechanisms of visual guidance of hand action in the parietal cortex of the monkey'. In Cerebral Cortex, 5, pp. 429–438.

SCHIEBER, M.H., POLIAKOV, A.V. (1998), 'Partial activation of the primary motor cortex hand area: effects of individuated movements'. In Journal of Neuroscience, 18, pp. 9038–9054.

SCHIENLE, A., STARK, R., WALKER, B., BLECKER, C., OTT, U., KIRSCH, P., SAMMER, G., VAITI, D. (2002), 'The insula is not specifically involved in disgust processing: an fMRI study'. In Neuroreport, 13, pp. 2023–2036.

SCHNEIDER, E.G. (1969), 'Two visual systems'. In Science, 163, pp. 895–902.

SCOTT, T.R., PLATA-SALAMAN, C.R., SMITH, V.L., GIZA, B.K. (1991), 'Gustatory neural coding in the monkey cortex: stimulus intensity'. In Journal of Neurophysiology, 65, pp. 76–86.

SELTZER, B., PANDYA, Y. (1994), 'Parietal temporal and occipital projections to cortex of the superior temporal sulcus in the rhesus monkey: a retrograde trace study'. In The Journal of Comparative Neurology, 243, pp. 445–463.

SEYAL, M., MULL, B., BHULLAR, N., AHMAD, T., GAGE, B. (1999), 'Anticipation and execution of a simple reading task enhance corticospinal excitability'. In Nature Reviews Neuroscience, 2, pp. 661–670.

SHIKATA, E., TANAKA, Y., NAKAMURA, H., TAIRA, M., SAKATA, H. (1996), 'Selectivity of the parietal visual neurons in 3D orientation of surface of stereoscopic stimuli'. In Neuroreport, 7, pp. 2389–2394.

SHOWERS, M.J.C., LAUER, E.W. (1961), 'Somatovisceral motor patterns in the insula'. In The Journal of Comparative Neurology, 117, pp. 107–115.

SINGER, T., SEYMUR, B., O'DOHERTY, J., KAUBE, H., DOLAN, R.J., FRITH, C.D. (2004), 'Empathy for pain involves the affective but not the sensory components of pain'. In Science, 303, pp. 1157–1162.

SMALL, D.M., GREGORY, M.D., MAK, Y.E., GITELMAN, D., MESULAM, M.M., PARRISH, T. (2003), 'Dissociation of neural representation of intensity and affective valuation in human gustation'. In Neuron, 39, pp. 701–711.

SPERRY, R.W. (1952), 'Neurology and the mind-brain problem'. In American Scientist, 40, pp. 291–312.

SPRENGELMEYER, R., RAUSCH, M., EYSEL, U.T., PRZUNTEK, H. (1998), 'Neural structures associated with recognition of facial expressions of basic emotions'. In Proceedings of Royal Society of London Series B Biological Sciences, 265, pp. 1927–1931.

STEIN, J.F. (1992), 'The representation of egocentric space in the posterior parietal cortex'. In The Behavorial and Brain Sciences, 15, pp. 691–700.

STERN, D.N. (1985), The interpersonal world of the infant. New York.

SWADESH, M. (1972), The Origin and Diversification of Language. Routledge & Kegan Paul, London.

TAIRA, M., MINE, S., GEORGOPULOS, A.P., MURATA, A., SAKATA, H. (1990), 'Parietal cortex neurons of the monkey related to the visual guidance of hand movement'. In Experimental Brain Research, 83, pp. 29–36.

TANIJ, J. (1994), 'The supplementary motor area in the cerebral cortex'. In Neuroscience Research, 19, pp. 251–268.

TANNÉ, J., BOUSSAOUD, D., BOYERZELLER, N., ROUILLER, E.M. (1995), 'Direct visual pathways for reaching movements in the macaque monkeys'. In Neuroreport, 7, pp. 267–272.

TANNER, J.E., BYRNE, R.W. (1996), 'Representation of action through iconic gesture in a captive lowland gorilla'. In Current Anthropology, 37, pp. 162–173.

TOBIAS, P.V. (1987), 'The brain of Homo habilis: a new level of organization in cerebral evolution'. In Journal of Human Evolution, 16, pp. 741–761.

TOKIMURA, H., TOKIMURA, Y., OLIVIERO, A., ASAKURA, T., ROTHWELL, J.C. (1996), 'Speech-induced changes in corticospinal excitability'. In Annual of Neurology, 40, pp. 628–634.

TOMASELLO, M., CALL, J. (1997), Primate Cognition. Oxford University Press, Oxford.

TOMASELLO, M., CALL, J., WARREN, J., FROST, G.T., CARPENTER, M., NAGEL, K. (1997), 'The ontogeny of chimpanzee gestural signals: a comparison across groups and generations'. In Evolution of Communication, 1, pp. 223–259.

TREVARTHEN, C.B. (1968), 'Two mechanisms of vision in primates'. In Psychologische Forschung, 31, pp. 299–337.

UMILTÀ, M.A., KOHLER, E., GALLESE, V., FOGASSI, L., FADIGA, L., KEYSERS, C., RIZZOLATTI, G. (2001), 'I know what you are doing: a neurophysiological study'. In Neuron, 32, pp. 91–101.

UNGERLEIDER, L., MISHKIN, M. (1982), 'Two cortical visual systems'. In INGLE, D.J., GOODALE, M.A., MANSFIELD, R.J.W. (editors), Analysis of Visual Behavior. MIT Press, Cambridge (MA), pp. 549–586.

VAN HOOF, J.A.R.A.M. (1962), 'Facial expressions in higher primates'. In Symposium of the Zoological Society of London, pp. 97–125.

VAN HOOF, J.A.R.A.M. (1967), 'The facial displays of the catarrhine monkeys and apes'. In MORRIS, D. (editor), Primate Ethology. Weidenfield & Nicholson, London, pp. 7–68.

VISALBERGHI, E., FRAGASZY, D. (1990), 'Do monkeys ape?'. In PARKER, S.T., GIBSON K.R. (editor), 'Language' and Intelligence in Monkeys and Apes. Cambridge University Press, Cambridge, pp. 247–273.

VISALBERGHI, E., FRAGASZY, D. (2002), 'Do monkeys ape? Ten years after'. In DAUTENHAHN, K., NEHANIV, C. (editors), Imitation in Animals and Artifacts, MIT Press, Boston (MA), pp. 471–499.

VOLPE, B.T., LEDUOUX, J.E., GAZZANIGA, M.S. (1979), 'Information processing of visual stimuli in an "extinguished" field'. In Nature, 282, p. 722.

VUILLEMIEUR, P., VALENZA, N., MAYER, E., REVERDIN, A., LANDIS, T. (1998), 'Near and far space in unilateral neglect'. In Annals of Neurology, 43, pp. 406–410.

VYGOTSKIJ, L.S. (1934), Thought and Language. MIT Press, Cambridge (MA) p 66.

WATKINS, K.E., STRAFELLA, A.P., PAUS, T. (2003), 'Seeing and hearing speech excites the motor system involved in speech production'. In Neurophysiologia, 41, pp. 989–994.

WEINRICH, M., WISE, S.P. (1982), 'The premotor cortex of the monkey'. In Journal of Neuroscience, 2, pp. 1329–1345.

WELFORD, A.T. (1968), Fundamentals of Skill. Methuen, London.

WICKER, B., KEYSERS, C., PLAILLY, J., ROVET, J.P., GALLESE, V., RIZZOLATTI, G. (2003), 'Both of us disgusted in my insula: the common neural basis of seeing and feeling disgust'. In Neuron, 40, pp. 655–664.

WISE, S.P., BOUSSAOUD, D., JOHNSON, P.B., CAMINITI, R. (1997), 'Premotor and parietal cortex: corticocortical connectivity and combinatorial computations'. In Annual Reviews of Neuroscience, 20, pp. 25–42.

WOHLSCHLÄGER, A., GATTIS, M., BEKKERING, H. (2003), 'Action generation and action perception in imitation: an instance of ideomotor principle'. In Philosophical Transactions of Royal Society of London Series B Biological Sciences, 358, pp. 501–515.

WOOLSEY, C.N. (1958), 'Organization of somatic sensory and motor areas of the cerebral cortex'. In HARLOW, H.F., WOOLSEY, C.N. (editor), Biological and Biochemical Bases of Behavior. University of Wisconsin Press, Madison (WI) pp. 63–81.

WOOLSEY, C.N., SETTLAGE, P.H., MEYER, D.R., SENCER, W., PINTO HAMUY, T., TRAVIS, A.M. (1952), 'Patterns of localization in precentral and 'supplementary' motor areas and their relation to the concept of a premotor area'. In Research publications - Association for Research in Nervous and Mental Disease, 30, pp. 238–264.

WUNDT, W. (1916), Elements of Folk Psychology. Engl. Trans. MacMillan, New York 1921.

YAXLEY, S., ROLLS, E.T., SIENKIEWICZ, Z.J. (1990), 'Gustatory responses of single neurons in the insula of macaque monkey'. In Journal of Neurophysiology, 63, pp. 689–700.

YOKOCHI, H., TANAKA, M., KUMASHIRO, M., IRIKI, A. (2003), 'Inferior parietal somatosensory neurons coding face-hand coordination in Japanese macaques'. In Somatosensory & Motor Research, 20, pp. 115–125.

ZAHN-WAXLER, C., RADKE-YARROW, M., WAGNER, E., CHAPMAN, M. (1992), 'Development of concern of others'. In Developmental Psychology, 28, pp. 126–136.

ZALD, D.H. (2003), 'The human amygdala and the emotional evaluation of sensory stimuli'. In Brain Research Reviews, 41, pp. 88–123.

ZALD, D.H., PARDO, J.V. (1997), 'Emotion, olfaction, and the human amygdala: amygdale activation during aversive olfactory stimulation'. In Proceedings of National Academy of Sciences of the United States of America, 94, pp. 4119–4124.

ZALD, D.H., PARDO, J.V. (2000), 'Functional neuroimaging of the olfactory system in humans'. In International Journal of Psychophysiology, 36, pp. 165–181.

ZALD, D.H., DONNDELINGER, M.J., PARDO, J.V. (1998a), 'Elucidating dynamic brain interactions with across-subjects correlational analyses of positron emission tomographic data: the functional connectivity of the amygdala and orbitofrontal cortex during olfactory tasks'. In Journal of Cerebral Blood Flow Metabolism, 18, pp. 896–905.

ZALD, D.H., LEE, J.T., FLUEGEL, K.W., PARDO, J.V. (1998b), 'Aversive gustatory stimulation activates limbic circuits in humans'. In Brain, 121, pp. 1143–1154.

ZIPSER, D., ANDERSEN, R.A. (1988), 'A back propagation programmed network that simulates response properties of a subset of posterior parietal neurons'. In Nature, 331, pp. 679–684

Index

Note: page numbers in *italics* refer to Figures.